THE ULTIMATE DUKAN DIET COOKBOOK FOR BEGINNERS

Nourishing Recipes for Weight Loss, Preserving Lean Muscle Mass, Blood Sugar Regulation, and Healthy Living

Steve Bryant, MD, RD

Copyright Page

Table of Contents

Introduction

The Dukan diet plan calls for cutting back on carbohydrates and fats while upping protein consumption. It promotes regular exercise and a diet heavy on whole, unprocessed foods rather than processed ones.

One hundred items that are permissible on the Dukan diet may be found on the official website. A total of 68 items are classified as "pure proteins," while 32 serve as veggies. In the final phases of a diet, a person might start introducing new foods.

Foods that are lean and packed with protein usually have less calories.

Consuming protein can satiety people because the process of digesting it requires more energy, leading to a little increase in caloric expenditure. Following a carbohydrate and fat restriction regimen, like the Atkin diet, puts the body into a famine state and compels it to use its fat stores as energy.

There are a few key ways in which the Dukan diet differs from the Atkins diet, another well-known HPLC. In order to stay hydrated on the Dukan diet, it is recommended that you consume 1.5 quarts (1.5 L) of water daily. Renal issues are common with HPLC diets, but according to Dukan, this will help avoid them. Additionally, there is a specific amount of oat bran that dieters must consume daily according to the Dukan diet. This, along with the recommended amount of water, may assist dieters who suffer from constipation on other HPLC regimens. In contrast to other high-protein low-carbohydrate diets, the Dukan regimen prohibits fatty foods like bacon and instead promotes lean protein sources.

Diet soft drinks, teas, nonfat milk, and a few other nonfat dairy items are permitted throughout the Dukan diet, as are artificial sweeteners (but no sugar). Additionally, it suggests flavoring with herbs, spices, onions, shallots, vinegar, and anything else that is low in calories and fat. If dieters are having trouble staying on track, these can help spice up the permitted high-protein meals so that they don't get bored with what they can eat. Even more stringent than the Atkins diet is the Dukan regimen. In the beginning, you may have only a little quantity of oat bran for carbs. Even vegetables like cabbage and spinach, which are low in carbohydrates, are off-limits. Additionally, there is a strict fat restriction and forbidden items including eggs, steaks, and chops, in contrast to the Atkins diet.

In its original form, the low-carbohydrate diet was known as the *Je ne sais pas maigrir* I do not know how to lose weight diet in France. The program was rebranded as the Dukan diet in 2010 when it made it to the UK, honoring its creator Pierre Dukan.

Chapter 1: Demystifying the Dukan Diet?

French physician Pierre Dukan created the widely followed *Dukan Diet*. A high-protein, low-carbohydrate diet is the foundation of this plan, which aims to help people lose weight quickly. The four stages of the diet are as follows: Attack, Cruise, Consolidation, and Stabilization.

Lean protein and limitless non-starchy veggies are the mainstays of the Attack Phase diet, which normally spans two to seven days. Inducing ketosis, a metabolic state in which the body burns fat for fuel, is the goal of this phase, which aims to jumpstart weight reduction.

After that comes the Cruise Phase, when participants switch it up by eating only protein some days and protein mixed with veggies that aren't starchy other days. This step keeps on till you reach your goal weight.

Reintroducing carbs and fats to the diet gradually during the Consolidation Phase helps to avoid rebound weight gain. This stage lasts around five days for every pound that was dropped in the first two.

At last, in the Stabilization Phase, you'll learn how to keep the weight off for good with a healthy diet and consistent exercise.

Some people think the Dukan Diet is too restrictive and might cause people to lose important nutrients or develop unhealthy eating habits. On top of that, there are health professionals that warn against eating too much animal protein in the long run. Talking to a doctor before beginning any diet is a good idea, but it's especially important if you have preexisting health concerns.

A Look at the History and Evolution of the Dukan Diet

French physician Pierre Dukan created the Dukan Diet in the '70s. The diet was first developed by Dr. Dukan to help his patients who were battling obesity and its related health problems. He developed a regimen that emphasized lean protein and minimized carbs and fats by drawing on his medical training and the high-protein diets of his ancestors.

Initially, the Dukan Diet was most successful in France, Dr. Dukan's home country. But 2000 saw a meteoric rise in its prominence when Dr. Dukan's book, *The Dukan Diet,* outlining the program's tenets and stages, was published. International interest in the diet was sparked when the book became a success in France and was subsequently translated into numerous languages.

Some changes and improvements were made to the Dukan Diet as it became popular across the world. Dr. Dukan kept improving his method by listening to his followers and incorporating new information on nutrition. Consistent with its original intent, the diet included four stages of eating meals that were both low in carbohydrates and high in protein.

Many people, including health professionals, nutritionists, and the general public, have strong opinions on the Dukan Diet. Proponents of the program say it helps people lose weight quickly and like the regimented approach it takes to eating. However, naysayers point out the diet's limitations, possible nutritional imbalances, and sustainability issues.

Regardless of the debates, the Dukan Diet changed the face of weight loss forever. There have been many conversations regarding the importance of macronutrients in good eating, and this diet plan has impacted other popular programs due to its focus on controlling portions and protein. Even if the Dukan Diet's star may have faded, it is still an influential nutritional framework that has left an indelible mark on the industry and the way people talk about food today.

Why the Dukan Diet is the Perfect Solution

For several reasons, the Dukan Diet has made a big splash in the world of diets and weight loss. First, it has given those who want a specific plan to follow a method that is both organized and easy to understand how to lose weight. The diet's four-stage method makes it easy for anybody to lose weight by providing a clear road map that prioritizes meals that are high in protein and low in carbohydrates.

A key component of the Dukan Diet is lean protein, which can aid in promoting fullness and maintaining muscle mass while dieters lose weight. The diet promotes nutrient-dense meals that increase feelings of fullness and satisfaction by highlighting protein-rich foods such as lean meats, fish, and tofu. This may help individuals avoid snacking in between meals or overeating.

In addition, the Dukan Diet can assist in the development of improved eating habits and an awareness of portion sizes through its emphasis on portion control and the progressive reintroduction of foods during the Consolidation Phase. Rather than depending on rigorous calorie tracking or restriction, this component of the diet encourages long-term weight control by encouraging mindful eating and moderation.

In addition, discussions over the importance of macronutrients in weight reduction and general health have been ignited by the Dukan Diet. Nutritionists and academics are investigating the pros and cons of this diet plan since it goes against the grain of traditional thinking by focusing on protein and limiting carbs. The effects of various eating habits on metabolic health and weight management are being better understood thanks to this continuing discussion.

Although the Dukan Diet has been the subject of controversy and criticism, its continued success shows how important it is among weight control plans. Although it might not work for everyone, those who are trying to lose weight and get healthier should consider it because of the methodical approach, the concentration on protein-rich meals, and the emphasis on small, lasting improvements. It is important to use caution while starting the Dukan Diet and to talk to a doctor before making any major adjustments to your diet, as is the case with any diet.

Chapter 2: Understanding the Principles and Phases of the Diet

apid weight loss with preserved muscle mass and general health is the goal of the Dukan Diet. Lean protein sources and non-starchy veggies take center stage in the diet's emphasis on low-carb, high-protein meals. In order to achieve rapid and substantial weight reduction, the diet emphasizes these nutrient-dense meals in an effort to put the body into a state of ketosis, when fat is burned for fuel.

The eating plan is divided into four parts, or stages, with its own set of rules and goals. During the first two to seven days, called the Attack Phase, you should eat mostly lean proteins such chicken, fish, eggs, and tofu. By cutting out carbs and resetting the body's metabolism to burn fat, this stage speeds up the weight reduction process.

The Cruise Phase follows the Attack Phase and consists of days when participants consume only protein and days when they consume protein along with non-starchy veggies. The alternating pattern maintains a healthy nutritional balance while continuing to stimulate weight reduction and fat burning throughout this phase, which continues until the goal weight loss is reached.

After participants achieve their weight reduction goals, they go on to the Consolidation Phase, where they work to maintain their new weight and avoid regaining it. In this stage, participants eat more carbs and fats again, but they still focus on getting enough lean protein and veggies. They do this by adding things like whole grains, fruits, cheese, and healthy fats to their diet.

Last but not least, the Dukan Diet contains a lifelong maintenance plan called the Stabilization Phase. During this stage, participants are motivated to maintain a healthy lifestyle by embracing a balanced diet that moderately includes all food groups. They are also encouraged to engage in regular physical exercise. To ensure long-term success and general health, this phase focuses on maintaining the new weight and preventing future weight return.

The Dukan Diet is a methodical and organized way to lose weight, with an emphasis on low-carbohydrate, high-protein meals that lead to quick and long-lasting benefits. The diet's concentration on nutrient-dense meals and straightforward rules make it a popular choice for those seeking to reduce weight and enhance their general health, while it might not work for everyone.

Phase 1: Attack

Inducing ketosis is the primary goal of the Attack Phase, the initial stage of the Dukan Diet, which aims to initiate quick weight reduction. Depending on the person's weight loss objectives, this stage might last anywhere from two to seven days. Pure protein, preferably from lean sources such chicken, fish, shellfish, eggs, and tofu, is what participants are told to eat throughout the Attack Phase.

Cutting up carbs during the Attack Phase is a great way to deplete your body's glycogen reserves and shift your metabolism to use fat for energy instead. Participants can get a head start on their weight reduction quest and see substantial immediate improvements by consuming just protein-rich meals.

There are no limits on the number of meals or the amount that participants can consume during the Attack Phase; participants are only allowed to eat until they are full. So long as you stick to the basic premise of eating only protein-rich meals, you may be flexible with your meal planning.

Some people, especially those used to diets strong in carbohydrates, may find the Attack Phase difficult, despite its effectiveness for quick weight reduction. As your body readjusts to a diet low in sugar and starches, you may experience typical withdrawal symptoms including lethargy, headaches, and an overwhelming desire for carbs during this time.

Despite its difficulties, the Attack Phase motivates participants to stay on the Dukan Diet and kick starts weight reduction, laying the groundwork for success in subsequent phases. The foundation it lays for the rest of the diet is vital if you want to succeed in the long run at managing your weight and improving your health.

Duration and Purpose

The Attack Phase, the first stage of the Dukan Diet, usually lasts anywhere from two to seven days, depending on the person's starting weight and weight reduction objectives. Inducing quick weight loss is the main goal of the Attack Phase, which involves cutting off carbs and eating just protein to kick start the body's fat-burning mechanism.

During this stage, it is recommended that individuals stay away from carbs, sweets, and fats while eating lean protein sources including chicken, fish, eggs, and tofu. Rapid weight reduction can be achieved by consuming just protein-rich meals. This puts the body into a state of ketosis, when it starts burning stored fat for energy.

Participants on the Dukan Diet get instant gratification and inspiration during the Attack Phase, the first and most important stage in their weight loss quest. It helps to get the metabolism going, control cravings, and set the stage for success in the rest of the diet with its short duration and rigorous rules.

By encouraging muscle maintenance and focusing on fat storage for energy, the Attack Phase lays the groundwork for long-term weight reduction success. This guarantees that dieters will experience rapid weight loss while also keeping their metabolic rate and body composition in a healthy range.

Phase 1 of the Dukan Diet can last anywhere from a few weeks to a few months, depending on the person, their starting weight, and their weight loss objectives. Regardless of how long it lasts, its main goal is the same: to help you lose weight quickly and keep it off by eating a lot of protein.

Allowed Foods

In the first stage of the Dukan Diet, called the Attack Phase, participants can eat a restricted variety of meals, with an emphasis on items high in pure protein. Because they are rich in protein and low in carbs, these foods are perfect for those who want to lose weight quickly by entering ketosis. Thin meats like turkey, thin cuts of beef, and pork tenderloin are among the items that can be eaten during Phase 1.

Salmon, tuna, shrimp, and lobster are among the seafood options available to participants, in addition to meats. Participants are free to try new flavors and cooking techniques with these protein-rich alternatives as long as they stick to the Phase 1 criteria.

As a flexible and easy-to-carry protein source, eggs are another mainstay item that is permissible during Phase 1. Eggs, whether eaten raw, cooked, or cooked into an omelet, are a great way to bulk up on protein at mealtimes and snacks, which can lead to sustained satiety.

Phase 1 of the Dukan Diet allows soy-based goods, including tofu, for people who are following a plant-based or vegetarian diet. For those who choose not to consume animal products or have dietary limitations, these alternatives provide a good amount of protein.

During Phase 1 of the Dukan Diet, you can eat a variety of meals that are carefully chosen to give you all the nutrients you need while also encouraging you to lose weight quickly by eating protein. Dieters may get a head start on losing weight and setting themselves up for success in subsequent phases by consuming lean proteins, seafood, eggs, and plant-based alternatives, such as tofu.

Phase 2: Cruise

After the first Attack Phase, the Dukan Diet moves on to the Cruise Phase, which is aimed at maintaining weight reduction while adding more variety to the diet. Phase 1's emphasis on pure protein makes for an unbalanced and unsustainable weight reduction strategy. The Cruise Phase, on the other hand, permits participants to combine lean protein sources with non-starchy veggies.

On days when they eat nothing but protein, or days when they eat protein with non-starchy veggies, participants in the Cruise Phase switch it up. While staying true to the Dukan Diet's fundamental principles, this alternate pattern gives you more leeway when organizing your meals. Vegetables like peppers, tomatoes, broccoli, spinach, and cucumbers can help people lose weight by adding flavor, texture, and nutrients to their meals.

Participants in the Cruise Phase often switch it up between days of eating nothing but protein and days of eating protein and vegetables until they reach their goal weight. By providing a wide range of foods and meal combinations, this method serves to both stimulate the metabolism and stave against monotony and boredom.

The Cruise Phase excels at fostering long-term commitment and sustainability, which is one of its main advantages. In order to set the groundwork for effective weight maintenance in the latter phases of the Dukan Diet, participants can acquire healthier eating habits and a better awareness of portion sizes by progressively adding non-starchy vegetables into their diet.

At its core, the Dukan Diet's Cruise Phase is a loosening up of restrictions after the rigorousness of Phase 1. Participants can maintain a stable weight reduction rate while eating more varied and satisfying meals by adding non-starchy veggies with lean protein sources.

Duration and Purpose

Phase 2 of the Dukan Diet, called the Cruise Phase, is all on losing weight in a sustainable way and is noted for its flexibility. In the Cruise Phase, participants are introduced to non-starchy veggies and lean protein sources, adding variety and nutrients to their meals, in contrast to the Attack Phase, which mainly focuses on protein consumption. The duration of this phase might vary based on the individual's development and weight reduction objectives, but it usually lasts until the desired results are reached.

During the Cruise Phase, you'll eat a larger variety of meals while still trying to lose weight. The metabolic state of ketosis achieved in Phase 1 may be maintained and the additional nutrients and fiber from vegetables can be enjoyed by participants by alternating between days of pure protein and days of protein mixed with vegetables. This method is great for maintaining an active metabolism, which in turn helps to avoid weight reduction plateaus and encourages consistent development.

The Cruise Phase also places a strong focus on long-term commitment and sustainability. Healthy eating habits, including portion control and balanced nutrition, can be achieved by progressively restoring non-starchy vegetables to the diet. This ensures that participants are prepared to retain their results over time and sets the stage for effective weight management in the following phases of the Dukan Diet.

Phase 2 lasts for different amounts of time depending on things including beginning weight, weight reduction objectives, and how far along the journey is. But its goal hasn't changed: to encourage long-term weight loss by dietary diversity and sustainability. Incorporating non-starchy veggies and lean protein sources allows participants to lose weight in a balanced and gratifying way, which is good for their health and the long run.

Food Options

After the Attack Phase, when participants were limited to protein exclusively, the Dukan Diet's second phase, the Cruise Phase, allowed them to eat a far larger variety of foods. At this point, the participants' protein intake will alternate between days when they eat only protein and days when they eat protein with non-starchy veggies. Incorporating more food diversity into the diet plan without sacrificing its weight reduction goals is a win-win.

Phase 2 meal choices include lean protein, a mainstay of the Dukan Diet. People taking part can keep eating lean meats including turkey, chicken breast, lean beef, and pork tenderloin. Participants may maintain satiety and muscle mass all day long with the aid of these protein sources, which also supply vital nutrients.

Aside from lean meats, Phase 2 participants are also allowed to eat shellfish and fish. Salmon, tuna, shrimp, and lobster are just a few options that provide flavor, diversity, and essential nutrients like omega-3 fatty acids. You may cook these seafood options in a variety of ways to suit your preferences, and they provide variety to the diet.

Adding nutrients, fiber, and volume to meals without significantly increasing carbs or calories is the goal of non-starchy veggies, which are an important part of Phase 2. On protein-and-vegetable days, load up on colorful, texturally and flavorfully rich vegetables like spinach, broccoli, tomatoes, cucumbers, peppers, and lettuce. They'll make your meals seem more complete and satiating.

The second phase of the Dukan Diet focuses on eating healthily and losing weight by balancing different nutrient-dense foods. Participants may have a diverse and enjoyable diet while still losing weight if they include lean proteins, seafood, and non-starchy veggies in their meals.

Phase 3: Consolidation

The third stage of the Dukan Diet, called the Consolidation Phase, is when dieters ease off on the rigid food restrictions of the first two stages. Phase 3 is where you keep the weight off for good, after you've lost a lot of it quickly in Phases 1 and

2. The Consolidation Phase involves easing back into carbs and lipids while maintaining an emphasis on lean protein and veggies that aren't starchy.

Fruits, starchy veggies, healthy grains, cheese, and dessert are once again within participants' purview during "celebration meals," which are a cornerstone of the Consolidation Phase's dietary restrictions. The frequency of these celebratory meals will grow from once a week to twice a week as the period goes on. Still emphasizing moderation and amount management, this method aids in avoiding deprivation emotions and fostering a positive connection with food.

Just like in the Attack Phase, a pure protein day must be maintained once a week throughout the

Consolidation Phase. To help with weight management and avoid rebound weight gain, this is a helpful reminder to focus on lean protein sources and to keep your metabolism in ketosis.

During the Consolidation Phase, patients are also urged to make physical activity a regular part of their lives, with the goal of engaging in moderate exercise for at least 30 minutes per day. This not only improves the diet's calorie-burning potential, but it also helps with general health and wellness.

When it comes to making the switch from losing weight to keeping it off, the Dukan Diet's Consolidation Phase offers a planned yet flexible approach. Participants may achieve a sustainable and healthy eating plan that promotes long-term success by easing back into carbs and lipids while maintaining an emphasis on lean protein and non-starchy veggies.

Duration and Purpose

A pivotal shift from active weight reduction to weight maintenance occurs during Phase 3 of the Dukan Diet, which is called the Consolidation Phase. The amount of time spent in this phase is usually proportional to the weight dropped thus far; as a rule of thumb, it's five days for every pound lost. In Phase 3, you'll aim to progressively include a broader range of foods back into your diet while sustaining the weight reduction and health improvements you've already made.

As they ease back into carbs, fruits, and dairy during the Consolidation Phase, participants are advised to keep lean protein, non-starchy veggies, and good eating practices as their top priorities. In order to avoid a quick return to pre-diet weights, this method of reintroduction helps people adjust to a healthier, more long-term eating routine.

In Phase 3, individuals are allowed to moderately indulge in their favorite foods during *celebration meals*, which are a significant component. In addition to teaching the value of moderation and quantity management, these meals offer a feeling of independence and flexibility. Participants may foster a healthy connection with food by integrating celebratory meals into their routine, which allows them to enjoy special events without feeling restricted or guilty.

In Phase 3, it's crucial to keep up with the regular exercise and healthy behaviors you started in

Phases 1 and 2. Maintaining an active lifestyle is highly encouraged, with participants being urged to exercise regularly and make thoughtful decisions regarding diet and portion sizes. Not only does this aid in the maintenance of weight and general health over the long run, but it also offers supplementary advantages including better cardiovascular health and stress management.

Consolidating success made in earlier stages and shifting to a sustainable and balanced eating habit are the overarching goals of Phase 3 of the Dukan Diet. Phase 3 aids participants in maintaining their weight reduction and achieving their long-term health and wellness objectives by progressively reintroducing a larger variety of foods and sustaining good habits.

Gradual Reintroduction of Foods

Participants progressively reintroduce items that were prohibited during earlier phases of the Dukan Diet during the Consolidation Phase. The goal of this broad reintroduction of foods is to help people go from losing weight actively to maintaining their weight, all the while giving them the framework they need to avoid a quick return to their original weight. Because it establishes the foundation for continued success and sustainability throughout the diet plan, it is an essential component.

The return of carbs, fruits, dairy, and other restricted food categories is an important part of the overall food reintroduction plan. The greater range of nutrients and tastes provided by these foods makes meal planning more fun and flexible, which in turn helps with weight control. It is recommended that participants ease into these meals by eating modest quantities and keeping track of their body's reaction to make sure they stay on track.

Along with the usual reintroduction of foods during the Consolidation Phase, there is also the idea of celebration meals. While still emphasizing the significance of moderation and quantity management, these meals provide participants the freedom to enjoy their favorite foods on occasion. Participants may foster a healthy connection with food by integrating celebratory meals into their routine, which allows them to enjoy special events without feeling restricted or guilty.

Participants are recommended to keep lean protein and non-starchy vegetables as their primary meal components during the general reintroduction of foods. Important for long-term weight control and general health, these meals supply necessary nutrients, make you feel full, and help you maintain your muscle mass.

When following the Dukan Diet, it is important to reintroduce foods gradually during the Consolidation Phase. This phase aims to help you eat more mindfully and in moderation. Maintaining weight reduction and improving health over the long run are both possible outcomes when individuals progressively reintroduce formerly limited meals while continuing to prioritize nutrient-dense alternatives.

Phase 4: Stabilization

At the end of the weight reduction journey, in Phase 4 of the Dukan Diet, which is called the Stabilization Phase, the focus shifts to long-term maintenance of the attained results. During this stage, you will learn how to make positive adjustments to your diet and way of life that will aid in your weight maintenance and general health. The previous stages had set durations and requirements; however, the Stabilization Phase is meant to be followed forever, with an emphasis on lifelong sustainable practices.

Maintaining the good eating habits developed in the prior diet stages is an important tenet of the

Stabilization Phase. In order to maintain a healthy diet, participants should limit their consumption of sugar, processed foods, and high-calorie snacks and increase their consumption of lean protein, fruits, vegetables, whole grains, and healthy fats. Maintaining a steady weight and general health are both aided by this well-rounded diet plan.

Making exercise a regular part of your routine is also crucial during the Stabilization Phase. To aid in weight maintenance and enhance health and fitness generally, participants are advised to exercise regularly, whether it's running, cycling, strength training, or brisk walking. Exercising on a regular basis has several health benefits, including lowering stress levels, improving cardiovascular health, and increasing metabolic rate.

Mindfulness and self-awareness are emphasized as important components of a healthy lifestyle throughout the Stabilization Phase of the Dukan Diet, alongside regular exercise and healthy nutrition. Paying attention to signs of hunger, controlling portion sizes, and making deliberate decisions on food and lifestyle behaviors are all things that participants are urged to do. Participants can prevent behaviors that lead to weight gain, such as emotional eating and overeating, by practicing mindfulness and self-awareness.

The Dukan Diet's Stabilization Phase is all about making a permanent change for the better in terms of your health and the amount of weight you lose. Participants can achieve long-term weight control and better health and well-being by adopting mindfulness into everyday living, frequent physical exercise, and appropriate eating habits.

Lifelong Guidelines

Guidelines for maintaining weight and general health are provided by the Dukan Diet for the whole of one's life, even after the diet's organized phases have ended. The long-term goal of these recommendations is to encourage a balanced lifestyle and the development of healthy behaviors.

The Dukan Diet stresses the need of lean protein as a meal base, which is one of its fundamental lifetime rules. Poultry, shellfish, low cuts of meat, tofu, and other lean protein sources are an important part of a healthy diet because they include necessary nutrients and help you feel full for longer. People can aid in the preservation of muscle mass, control their hunger, and maintain a healthy weight by eating meals that contain lean protein.

The Dukan Diet places an emphasis on lean protein and promotes the intake of vitamin-, mineral-, and fiber-rich non-starchy foods. These veggies boost health and satisfaction by adding bulk and nutrients to meals without significantly increasing calorie intake. A varied diet rich in colorful vegetables can help people maintain optimal health by providing them with a variety of nutrients and antioxidants.

Regular physical exercise is highly recommended as a vital part of a healthy lifestyle according to the

Dukan Diet, which is another lifetime recommendation. Exercising has several positive effects on health, including weight loss and maintenance, cardiovascular health, physical strength, and mental clarity. People may boost their fitness, lower their chance of developing chronic diseases, and improve their quality of life in general by making exercise a regular part of their routine.

Furthermore, being conscious and self-aware in relation to one's eating habits and lifestyle choices is emphasized upon by the Dukan Diet. A person may reduce their risk of weight gain by being aware of when they are hungry, controlling their portion sizes, and making deliberate choices regarding what they eat and how active they are. People may keep their weight and health in check and have a positive connection with food if they practice mindfulness and self-awareness.

The Dukan Diet is a way of life that encourages a healthy relationship with food, exercise, and mindfulness practices to help people maintain a healthy weight and quality of life throughout their lives. If people follow these rules on a regular basis, they will see improvements to their health that will continue for years.

Maintaining Weight Loss

Keeping off the weight you lose is no easy feat, but it is doable with the correct approach and frame of mind. Adopting habits that promote long-term weight management and general health is vital for persons who have successfully lost weight, whether it is through the Dukan Diet or another method.

Sticking to a healthy, well-balanced diet is an important part of keeping the weight off. To achieve this goal, one must consciously choose to eat less processed foods, sweets, and bad fats and more entire foods like lean protein, veggies, whole grains, and healthy fats. People can maintain a healthy weight by limiting their caloric intake and eating more nutrient-dense meals while watching their portions.

Keeping up with regular exercise is also essential for keeping the weight off. Physical activity has several health benefits, including boosting metabolism, increasing lean muscle mass, and enhancing general fitness and wellness. People are more likely to stick with their fitness routines and like them over the long haul if they find activities like walking, running, cycling, swimming, or strength training that they enjoy and can maintain.

In addition to physical activity and a balanced diet, people should work on improving their mental attitude toward food and their perception of their own body. This includes not being harsh or rigid with one's eating habits and instead being kind and compassionate with oneself. Individuals may better handle obstacles and keep their weight reduction progress going if they learn to cope with stress, emotions, and cravings.

Efforts to sustain weight reduction can be amplified by creating a supportive atmosphere. A great way to stay motivated, accountable, and encouraged is to surround yourself with others who share your health objectives, whether that's family, friends, or support groups. It might be simpler to remain on course and overcome hurdles when you have a support system in place.

It takes a mix of good eating habits, frequent exercise, a happy attitude, and a supportive environment to keep the weight off. People may enhance their health, energy, and quality of life in the long run by making lasting lifestyle adjustments and putting self-care first, which will help them keep the weight off.

Chapter 3: Dukan Diet Recipes

Recommended Dukan Diet Breakfast Recipes

Fruity Curry Chicken Salad

Ingredients

2 cups cooked chicken breast, diced

1/2 cup diced apple

1/2 cup halved grapes

1/4 cup chopped celery

1/4 cup chopped almonds

1/4 cup raisins

1/2 cup mayonnaise

1 tablespoon curry powder

Salt and pepper to taste

Method

In a large mixing bowl, combine the diced chicken, apple, grapes, celery, almonds, and raisins.

In a small bowl, mix together the mayonnaise and curry powder until well combined.

Pour the curry mayo over the chicken mixture and toss until everything is evenly coated.

Season with salt and pepper to taste.

Chill in the refrigerator for at least 30 minutes before serving.

Dutch Baby Pancakes

Ingredients

2 tablespoons butter

2 tablespoons brown sugar, packed

1/4 teaspoon cinnamon

1 cup apples, peeled or unpeeled, thinly sliced

2 eggs, large

1/2 cup flour

1/2 cup milk

1/4 teaspoon salt

Method

Heat the oven to 400°F.

Melt the butter in a 9" pie plate in the oven. Brush the butter on to the side of the pie plate. Sprinkle the brown sugar and 1/4 teaspoon ground cinnamon evenly over the melted butter in the plate. Arrange 1 cup of thinly sliced peeled or unpeeled baking apples over the brown sugar.

Now make the pancake batter by beating the eggs slightly in a medium bowl with a wire whisk or hand beater. Beat in the remaining ingredients, just until mixed. Do not over beat the mixture.

Pour the batter into the pie plate over top of the apples.

Bake for 30-35 minutes or until the pancake is puffy and deep golden brown. Invert the pancake on to a large plate so the apples are showing on the top. Serve it immediately, sprinkled with lemon juice and powdered sugar if desired.

Sesame Pasta Chicken Salad

Ingredients

2 cups cooked chicken breast, diced

2 cups cooked pasta (such as rotini or penne)

1/2 cup shredded carrots

1/2 cup sliced bell peppers (any color)

1/4 cup chopped green onions

1/4 cup sesame seeds

1/4 cup soy sauce

2 tablespoons rice vinegar

1 tablespoon sesame oil

1 tablespoon honey

Salt and pepper to taste

Method

In a large mixing bowl, combine the diced chicken, cooked pasta, shredded carrots, sliced bell peppers, green onions, and sesame seeds.

In a small bowl, whisk together the soy sauce, rice vinegar, sesame oil, and honey.

Pour the dressing over the chicken and pasta mixture and toss until well coated.

Season with salt and pepper to taste.

Chill in the refrigerator for at least 30 minutes before serving.

Chinese Chicken Salad

Ingredients

2 cups cooked chicken breast, shredded

4 cups shredded cabbage (Napa or regular)

1 cup shredded carrots

1/4 cup sliced almonds, toasted

1/4 cup chopped cilantro

1/4 cup chopped green onions

1/4 cup crispy chow mein noodles (optional)

1/4 cup soy sauce

2 tablespoons sesame oil

2 tablespoons rice vinegar

1 tablespoon honey

1 teaspoon grated ginger

1 clove garlic, minced

Method

In a large mixing bowl, combine the shredded chicken, shredded cabbage, shredded carrots, sliced almonds, chopped cilantro, and green onions.

In a small bowl, whisk together the soy sauce, sesame oil, rice vinegar, honey, grated ginger, and minced garlic to make the dressing.

Pour the dressing over the salad and toss until everything is evenly coated.

Chill in the refrigerator for at least 30 minutes before serving.

Sprinkle with crispy chow mein noodles before serving if desired.

Chicken Salad with Bacon, Lettuce, and Tomato

Ingredients

2 cups cooked chicken breast, diced

1/2 cup cooked bacon, crumbled

1 cup diced tomatoes

1 cup diced cucumber

1/2 cup diced red onion

2 cups chopped lettuce

1/4 cup mayonnaise

2 tablespoons chopped fresh parsley

1 tablespoon lemon juice

Salt and pepper to taste

Method

In a large mixing bowl, combine the diced chicken, crumbled bacon, diced tomatoes, diced cucumber, diced red onion, and chopped lettuce.

In a small bowl, whisk together the mayonnaise, chopped parsley, and lemon juice.

Pour the dressing over the chicken and vegetable mixture and toss until well combined.

Season with salt and pepper to taste.

Chill in the refrigerator for at least 30 minutes before serving.

Buffalo Chicken Pasta Salad

Ingredients

2 cups cooked chicken breast, diced or shredded

2 cups cooked pasta (such as penne or rotini)

1/2 cup diced celery

1/2 cup diced carrots

1/4 cup crumbled blue cheese

1/4 cup ranch dressing

1/4 cup buffalo sauce

Salt and pepper to taste

Optional: chopped green onions for garnish

Method

In a large bowl, combine the diced chicken, cooked pasta, diced celery, and diced carrots.

In a small bowl, mix together the ranch dressing and buffalo sauce until well combined.

Pour the dressing over the chicken and pasta mixture and toss until evenly coated.

Gently fold in the crumbled blue cheese.

Season with salt and pepper to taste.

Garnish with chopped green onions if desired.

Chill in the refrigerator for at least 30 minutes before serving.

Almond Chicken Salad

Ingredients

2 cups cooked chicken breast, diced

1/2 cup sliced almonds, toasted

1/2 cup diced celery

1/4 cup diced red onion

1/4 cup chopped fresh parsley

1/2 cup mayonnaise

2 tablespoons lemon juice

Salt and pepper to taste

Method

In a large bowl, combine the diced chicken, sliced almonds, diced celery, diced red onion, and chopped parsley.

In a small bowl, whisk together the mayonnaise and lemon juice until well combined.

Pour the dressing over the chicken and almond mixture and toss until evenly coated.

Season with salt and pepper to taste.

Chill in the refrigerator for at least 30 minutes before serving.

Parmesan and Basil Chicken Salad

Ingredients

2 cups cooked chicken breast, diced

1/4 cup grated Parmesan cheese

1/4 cup chopped fresh basil

1/4 cup diced red bell pepper

1/4 cup diced red onion

1/4 cup mayonnaise

2 tablespoons lemon juice

Salt and pepper to taste

Method

In a large bowl, combine the diced chicken, grated Parmesan cheese, chopped basil, diced red bell pepper, and diced red onion.

In a small bowl, whisk together the mayonnaise and lemon juice until well combined.

Pour the dressing over the chicken and herb mixture and toss until evenly coated.

Season with salt and pepper to taste.

Chill in the refrigerator for at least 30 minutes before serving.

Dijon Chicken Salad

Ingredients

2 cups cooked chicken breast, diced

1/2 cup diced apple

1/4 cup chopped walnuts

1/4 cup diced celery

1/4 cup dried cranberries

1/4 cup mayonnaise

2 tablespoons Dijon mustard

1 tablespoon lemon juice

Salt and pepper to taste

Method

In a large bowl, combine the diced chicken, diced apple, chopped walnuts, diced celery, and dried cranberries.

In a small bowl, whisk together the mayonnaise, Dijon mustard, and lemon juice until well combined.

Pour the dressing over the chicken and fruit mixture and toss until evenly coated.

Season with salt and pepper to taste.

Chill in the refrigerator for at least 30 minutes before serving.

Crunchy Cauliflower and Tomato Salad

Ingredients

1 head cauliflower, cut into small florets

1 cup cherry tomatoes, halved

1/4 cup sliced almonds, toasted

2 tablespoons chopped fresh parsley

2 tablespoons olive oil

1 tablespoon balsamic vinegar

Salt and pepper to taste

Method

Steam the cauliflower florets until tender but still crunchy. Drain and let cool.

In a large bowl, combine the cauliflower florets, cherry tomatoes, toasted sliced almonds, and chopped fresh parsley.

In a small bowl, whisk together the olive oil and balsamic vinegar to make the dressing.

Pour the dressing over the cauliflower and tomato mixture and toss until everything is well coated. Season with salt and pepper to taste.

Mediterranean Bean Salad

Ingredients

2 cups cooked beans (such as chickpeas, kidney beans, or cannellini beans), drained and rinsed

1 cucumber, diced

1 bell pepper, diced

1/4 cup chopped red onion

1/4 cup chopped fresh parsley

1/4 cup crumbled feta cheese

2 tablespoons olive oil

1 tablespoon red wine vinegar

1 teaspoon dried oregano

Salt and pepper to taste

Method

In a large bowl, combine the cooked beans, diced cucumber, diced bell pepper, chopped red onion, chopped fresh parsley, and crumbled feta cheese.

In a small bowl, whisk together the olive oil, red wine vinegar, dried oregano, salt, and pepper to make the dressing.

Pour the dressing over the bean salad and toss until everything is well coated.

Tomato and Egg Stir Fry

Ingredients

2 tablespoons vegetable oil

4 eggs, beaten

2 tomatoes, diced

2 cloves garlic, minced

1 tablespoon soy sauce

1 teaspoon sugar

Salt and pepper to taste

Chopped green onions for garnish (optional)

Method

Heat vegetable oil in a large skillet or wok over medium-high heat.

Pour the beaten eggs into the skillet and cook, stirring gently, until scrambled and set. Remove the scrambled eggs from the skillet and set aside.

In the same skillet, add diced tomatoes and minced garlic. Cook for 2-3 minutes, until the tomatoes start to soften.

Return the scrambled eggs to the skillet. Add soy sauce, sugar, salt, and pepper. Stir well to combine. Cook for another 2-3 minutes, stirring occasionally, until heated through.

Garnish with chopped green onions before serving, if desired.

Mini Frittatas with Quinoa

Ingredients

1 cup cooked quinoa

6 eggs

1/4 cup milk

1/2 cup diced bell pepper

1/4 cup chopped spinach

1/4 cup grated Parmesan cheese

Salt and pepper to taste

Cooking spray

Method

Preheat your oven to 375°F (190°C). Grease a mini muffin tin with cooking spray.

In a large bowl, whisk together eggs and milk until well combined.

Stir in cooked quinoa, diced bell pepper, chopped spinach, grated Parmesan cheese, salt, and pepper.

Spoon the egg mixture into the prepared mini muffin tin, filling each cup almost to the top.

Bake in the preheated oven for 12-15 minutes, or

until the frittatas are set and lightly golden on top.

Remove the mini frittatas from the muffin tin and

let cool slightly before serving.

Recommended Dukan Diet Lunch Recipes

Vegetable Quiche

Ingredients

1 cup Swiss cheese, grated

1/2 cup cheddar cheese, grated

2 cups vegetables, chopped (any or a mix of asparagus, red peppers, mushrooms, zucchini or yellow zucchini)

12 eggs

1 cup milk

1 cup heavy cream

1/2 teaspoon salt

1/4 teaspoon black pepper

1/4 teaspoon nutmeg, optional

Prepared pie crust is optional

Method

Preheat oven to 375ºF.

Spray a 12" quiche pan or a deep dish pie pan with non-stick spray. Spread cheese on the bottom of the pan. Add chopped vegetables. Whisk eggs, milk, cream and seasonings together. Pour over cheese and vegetables. Bake until just set in the middle, about 45 minutes.

Poached Italian Eggs

Ingredients

1 tablespoon olive oil

1/2 onion, chopped

1 clove garlic, chopped

28 ounce can tomatoes, diced or 1 bottle passata (strained tomatoes)

1 zucchini

1/2 teaspoon basil, dried, or 1 tablespoon fresh basil minced

Salt to taste

Freshly ground pepper to taste

6 to 8 eggs

2 tablespoons parsley, fresh, minced

Method

Heat the olive oil in a frying pan. Add the chopped onion and garlic and sauté until they are just soft. Cut the ends off the zucchini and slice it in half lengthwise. Slice the zucchini into fairly thin half-moons. Add them to the sauté pan and cook for about 3 or 4 minutes.

Add the tomatoes or tomato passata (see notes below) to the pan. Add the dried basil if you are using dried, plus salt and pepper to taste.

Cook for about 20 to 25 minutes, until the sauce has thickened. If you are using fresh minced basil add it now.

Crack the eggs right on to the sauce, making sure they are evenly spaced on the pan. Cover and cook the eggs for about 6 to 8 minutes over medium heat, until the whites are set but the yolks are still runny. (If you like your egg whites firm, cook the mixture for 2 minutes longer).

Sprinkle with the fresh minced parsley before serving.

Grilled Trout Recipe

Ingredients

3 pounds rainbow trout fillets

2 tablespoons butter

1 lemon

1/2 cup French dressing

Salt and pepper to taste

Method

Place the trout onto heavy aluminum foil. Dot with butter and squeeze the lemon on to the fish. Spread with salad dressing. Salt and pepper to taste (remember the salad dressing will have salt in it). Wrap the foil around the fish fillet and seal tightly. Place the trout "package" on a hot grill, on the side of a fire or in a 350ºF preheated oven. Cook for 10 to 15 minutes, until flaky. Exact cooking time depends on the thickness of the fish.

Remove fish from the foil and serve.

Rainbow Trout Amandine

Ingredients

2 pounds rainbow trout fillets

1 lemon, cut into 8 wedges

1/4 cup almonds, sliced and toasted

1/4 cup parsley, fresh, chopped

Method

Preheat the oven's broiler.

Lightly coat the rack of a broiler pan with nonstick cooking spray.

Rinse the fish and pat it dry. Rub the trout fillets with lemon juice from 2 of the lemon wedges. Place the fish on the broiler pan and broil for 3 to 5 minutes until it is almost done, turning once during cooking time. Broil about 4 to 5 inches from the heating element.

Sprinkle fish with almonds and broil for 1 or 2 minutes more, until the fish flakes with a fork. Sprinkle with the chopped parsley and serve with remaining lemon wedges.

Soba Noodle Salad Recipe

Ingredients

8 ounces soba noodles

1 1/2 teaspoons vegetable oil

10 mushrooms, sliced

1 onion, sliced

1 carrot, shaved or cut into thin julienne strips

1/2 red pepper, chopped

1 bunch spinach, or baby kale

1/4 cup water

2 cups bok choy, sliced

3 tablespoons teriyaki sauce

2 tablespoons rice vinegar

1 tablespoon dark sesame oil

2 cloves garlic, minced

2 teaspoons hoisin sauce

1/4 teaspoon Asian chili sauce

Method

Cook noodles in a large pot of boiling salted water for 6 to 8 minutes or until just tender. Be careful to not overcook the noodles. Drain and rinse under cold running water to cool. Place in a large bowl. Heat 1 1/2 teaspoons of oil in a large nonstick skillet over medium-high heat until hot. Add the mushrooms, onions, carrots and peppers and cook for five minutes or until tender. Place in the bowl with the noodles.

To the same skillet add the spinach and water. Cook for one to two minutes or until the spinach is just wilted, stirring constantly. Add the spinach to the bowl. Cook the bok choy, adding a little more water if necessary, for 2 to 3 minutes or until barely tender. Add the bok choy to the noodles and toss to combine.

In a medium bowl, whisk together all the vinaigrette ingredients. Pour over the salad and toss it all together well to combine.

Pastitsio

Ingredients

1 1/2 pounds ground beef

1 cup onion, chopped

1/4 cup tomato paste

1/3 cup water

1/4 cup beef stock, or dry red wine

1 teaspoon salt

1/4 teaspoon black pepper

1/4 teaspoon cinnamon

3/4 pound penne pasta, uncooked

1 tablespoon vegetable oil

3 tablespoons butter, melted

1 egg, beaten

1/4 cup half and half cream

8 ounces Parmesan cheese, grated

For the Cream Sauce:

1/4 cup butter

4 cups milk

4 tablespoons cornstarch

Salt to taste

5 eggs

Method

Preheat the oven to 350°F. Butter a 13"x9" baking dish and set it aside.

In a large skillet, brown the meat and onions, stirring often to break up the meat. Add tomato paste, 1/3 cup water, wine or beef broth, 1 teaspoon salt, pepper and cinnamon. Simmer for 10 minutes until the liquid evaporates.

Meanwhile, bring 2 to 3 quarts of water to a boil in a 5 quart pot or Dutch oven. Add 2 teaspoons of salt and 1 tablespoon of oil. Add the pasta, being sure that the water continues to boil. Cook the pasta uncovered until tender but firm, according to the directions on the package, stirring occasionally to make sure it stays separated. Drain the pasta. Pour the melted butter over the pasta, tossing it all together well. Set the pasta aside.

In a small bowl, stir together the egg and cream to blend together. Set aside 3 tablespoons Parmesan cheese for the topping. Toss the egg mixture and remaining cheese with the cooked pasta.

Place the pasta mixture into the prepared baking dish. Spread the meat sauce over the pasta and pour the creamy sauce over the meat sauce. Sprinkle with the remaining 3 tablespoons of cheese and bake in a preheated oven for 45 minutes or until top of the casserole is golden.

To Make the Cream Sauce:

In a medium saucepan, combine the butter, milk and cornstarch. Stir over low heat until thickened, about 15 minutes. Stir in the salt.

Remove from the heat. Beat the eggs together well and very slowly stir about 1 cup of the hot sauce into the beaten eggs. Do this very gradually to allow the eggs to warm slowly. Too quickly and the eggs will cook. Gradually add the egg mixture to the sauce and stir to blend it together. Makes about 5 cups of cream sauce.

Baked Salmon Fillet

Ingredients

12 spinach leaves, large

2 pounds salmon fillets, 4 fillets, or 2 pounds of whole salmon

1 tablespoon fresh dill, chopped

Salt & pepper to taste

1 cup cold water

1 1/2 teaspoons butter

2/3 cup green onions, sliced

1 clove garlic, minced

Method

Preheat oven to 325ºF.

Arrange spinach leaves on the bottom of a 13"x9" baking dish. Lay salmon on top. Sprinkle salmon with dill, salt and pepper. Mix water and butter together and pour it over the salmon. Top with green onions and garlic. Cover the baking dish tightly with foil.

Bake for 25 to 30 minutes, or until salmon flakes easily when tested with a fork, basting two or three times. Serve with the spinach and juices.

Crispy Baked Halibut

Ingredients

1 1/4 pounds halibut steaks, or thick fillets, fresh or frozen

2 teaspoons vegetable oil

3/4 cup bread crumbs, soft

2 tablespoons parmesan cheese, grated

1 tablespoon fresh tarragon, snipped or 1/2 teaspoon dried tarragon, crushed

1/2 teaspoon paprika

1 dash pepper

Fresh lemon wedges, for serving - optional

Method

Preheat oven to 450ºF.

Cut thawed fish into four portions. Pat dry and brush each portion with cooking oil.

In a shallow dish, stir together bread crumbs, parmesan cheese, tarragon, paprika and pepper.

Dip fish into crumb mixture to coat both sides.

Arrange pieces in a 12"x7 1/2" baking dish. Sprinkle any leftover crumb mixture on top. Bake fish at 450ºF, uncovered for 8 to 12 minutes in a hot oven, until fish flakes easily with a fork. Do not turn during baking. Serve with fresh lemon wedges for drizzling.

Lemon Dill Fish

Ingredients

1 pound fish fillets

1/2 cup Miracle Whip, or other similar salad dressing

2 tablespoons lemon juice

1/2 teaspoon lemon peel, grated

1 teaspoon dill

Method

Mix together Miracle Whip, juice, lemon peel and dill.

Grease grill or broil pan. Place fish on greased pan and brush with half of the sauce mixture.

Grill or broil about 5 to 8 minutes. Turn fish over and brush with the remaining sauce. Broil or grill for another 5 to 8 minutes, or until fish flakes easily with a fork.

Shrimp Scampi Recipe

Ingredients

1 pound raw shrimp, large, peeled and deveined

3 tablespoons butter, unsalted, softened

1/8 cup olive oil

4 - 6 cloves garlic, chopped

1 tablespoon lemon juice

1/4 cup white wine, optional - see Variations below

Salt and pepper to taste

1/4 cup parmesan cheese

Method

Place butter and oil into large sauté pan and heat to melt the butter. Add garlic and sauté for 1 minute. Add wine, lemon juice, salt and pepper, and the shrimp. Cook until shrimp turn opaque or pink, stirring occasionally. Stir in parmesan cheese before serving.

Tuna Noodle Casserole Recipe with Broccoli

Ingredients

8 ounces egg noodles

10 ounces broccoli, frozen

7 ounces canned tuna, flaked

10 1/2 ounces cream of chicken soup, canned

10 1/2 ounces cream of celery soup, canned

5 ounces milk, 1/2 of a soup can

1/2 cup potato chips, crushed, or crushed plain crackers

Method

Heat oven to 450°F.

Cook egg noodles. Drain and set aside. Cook broccoli about 3 minutes, then drain.

Mix together noodles, tuna, broccoli, the soups and milk in a large baking dish. Sprinkle the top with the crushed potato chips. Bake 30 minutes.

Salmon Patties Recipe

Ingredients

2 pounds potatoes, peeled and sliced

1 cup salmon, cooked, flaked and boned

1/2 cup haddock, cooked, flaked and boned (or use

1 1/2 cups salmon)

1 tablespoon ketchup

1 teaspoon Worcestershire sauce

Salt and freshly ground pepper

1 green onion, green part only, chopped

1/2 cup corn kernels, optional

1 tablespoon parsley, finely chopped

1 egg

Fat for deep frying

1 egg

2 tablespoons water

1 cup bread crumbs, dried

Lemon wedges

Method

Boil the potatoes until soft, then drain them and mash them (see hints below). It is important that the potato is free from lumps. Mix the flaked fish into the potatoes, gradually adding seasonings, onion and parsley. Add the corn if you are using it. Bind it together by mixing in the beaten egg.

Shape the mixture into patties. Put them onto a tray or cookie sheet and chill in the freezer or top of fridge for 30 minutes.

Flour your hands and dip each cake into the beaten egg mixed with water, and then coat with the bread crumbs. Press the crumbs well into the cakes. Chill for another 30 minutes.

Fry for about 4-5 minutes until crisp.

Serve with lemon wedges.

Scallop Sauté

Ingredients

1 pound sea scallops, washed and dried thoroughly

1/2 teaspoon salt

1/4 teaspoon paprika

1/8 teaspoon black pepper, freshly ground

1 clove garlic

1 tablespoon fresh parsley, finely chopped

3 tablespoons lemon juice

2 tablespoons butter

Method

Heat a large skillet generously coated with cooking spray over medium-high heat. Add the scallops and cook, stirring frequently, for 8 minutes, or until golden brown. Remove to a serving platter and keep warm.

In the same skillet, combine the lemon juice, butter, parsley, salt, paprika, pepper, and garlic. Cook, stirring until the butter is melted. Pour over the scallops.

Halibut Baked With Vegetables

Ingredients

2/3 cup onion, thinly sliced

1 pound halibut, or other similar meaty fish

1 yellow pepper, sliced

1 red pepper, sliced

1 cup mushrooms, sliced

1/4 cup fresh parsley, chopped

1/2 cup white wine

2 tablespoons lemon juice

Fresh dill

1/8 teaspoon pepper

Method

Preheat oven to 400ºF.

Arrange onion slices in the bottom of a baking dish sprayed with non-stick spray and place the fish on top. Combine the next four ingredients and spread over the fish. Combine wine, lemon juice, dill and pepper and pour over the whole thing.

Cover and bake for 20 minutes.

Serve with lemon wedges.

Baked Rice Pudding Recipe

Ingredients

1/2 cup long grain rice, uncooked

1 cup water

2 eggs, large

1/2 cup sugar

1/2 cup raisins, or chopped dried apricots, both optional

2 1/2 cups milk

1 teaspoon vanilla

1/4 teaspoon salt

1/2 teaspoon ground cinnamon, or nutmeg

Whipped cream, optional

Method

Heat the rice and water to boiling in a 1 1/2 quart saucepan, stirring once or twice. Reduce the heat to low. Cover and simmer for 14 minutes (do not lift the cover or stir). All the water should be absorbed.

Heat the oven to 325ºF.

Beat the eggs in an ungreased 1 1/2 quart casserole. Stir in the sugar, raisins or chopped dried apricots, milk, vanilla, salt and hot rice. Sprinkle with cinnamon.

Bake uncovered for 45 minutes, stirring every 5 or 10 minutes. When the cooking time is done the top of the pudding should be very wet and not set. Stir well. Let stand for 15 minutes. Enough liquid will be absorbed while standing to make the pudding creamy. Tops with extra cinnamon if desired.

Note that over baking may cause the pudding to curdle.

Serve warm or cover and refrigerate about 3 hours or until chilled.

Serve with whipped cream. Refrigerate any remaining pudding.

Recommended Dukan Diet Dinner Recipes

Macaroni Chicken Casserole

Ingredients

1/2 cup onion, chopped

3 tablespoons butter, melted

2 cans cream of chicken soup, undiluted

2 cups cheddar cheese, shredded

1 cup milk

3 1/2 cups cooked chicken, chopped

2 1/2 cups cooked macaroni, about 1 cup dry

1/4 cup cracker crumbs, buttery style is best

Method

Preheat oven to 350°F.

Sauté the onion in butter in a large skillet until tender. Add the soup and 1 1/2 cups of cheese. Gradually stir in the milk. Cook over medium heat until the cheese melts. Stir in the chicken and macaroni.

Pour the mixture into a greased 2 1/2 quart casserole. Sprinkle the top with the cracker crumbs.

Bake for 30 minutes or until thoroughly heated. Top with the remaining cheese and bake an additional 5 minutes.

Macaroni and Cheese Recipe

Ingredients

5 tablespoons butter, divided

3 tablespoons flour

2 1/2 cups whole milk

1 pound cheddar cheese, grated extra sharp

1/2 teaspoon dry mustard

Pinch cayenne pepper

Dash Worcestershire sauce

Salt and pepper to taste

1 pound elbow macaroni, uncooked

1/4 cup Parmesan cheese, grated

1/2 cup plain bread crumbs

Method

Preheat the oven to 350°F.

Using 1 tablespoon butter, generously grease a 2-quart baking dish.

Melt 3 tablespoons butter, add flour and cook over moderate heat for 2 minutes, stirring constantly. Do not brown.

Add milk and whisk constantly until thickened, 3 to 5 minutes. Add cheddar cheese and stir until it is well blended into the sauce. Add the seasonings and stir. Remove from the heat.

Meanwhile, cook the macaroni according to package directions. Drain well, but do not rinse. Put macaroni back into the pot and add the cheese sauce. Stir until it is all well mixed.

Pour the macaroni and cheese mixture into a baking dish, sprinkle with bread crumbs and Parmesan cheese and dot with pieces of the remaining tablespoon of butter.

Bake at 350°F for 30 minutes or until bubbling and golden brown. Let stand 10 to 15 minutes before serving.

Soba Noodle Salad

Ingredients

8 ounces soba noodles

1 1/2 teaspoons vegetable oil

10 mushrooms, sliced

1 onion, sliced

1 carrot, shaved or cut into thin julienne strips

1/2 red pepper, chopped

1 bunch spinach, or baby kale

1/4 cup water

2 cups bok choy, sliced

3 tablespoons teriyaki sauce

2 tablespoons rice vinegar

1 tablespoon dark sesame oil

2 cloves garlic, minced

2 teaspoons hoisin sauce

1/4 teaspoon Asian chili sauce

Method

Cook noodles in a large pot of boiling salted water for 6 to 8 minutes or until just tender. Be careful to not overcook the noodles. Drain and rinse under cold running water to cool. Place in a large bowl.

Heat 1 1/2 teaspoons of oil in a large nonstick skillet over medium-high heat until hot. Add the mushrooms, onions, carrots and peppers and cook for five minutes or until tender. Place in the bowl with the noodles.

To the same skillet add the spinach and water. Cook for one to two minutes or until the spinach is just wilted, stirring constantly. Add the spinach to the bowl. Cook the bok choy, adding a little more water if necessary, for 2 to 3 minutes or until barely tender. Add the bok choy to the noodles and toss to combine.

In a medium bowl, whisk together all the vinaigrette ingredients. Pour over the salad and toss it all together well to combine.

Cheese and Bacon with Noodle Casserole

Ingredients

6 to 8 slices bacon

8 ounces wide noodles, or pasta shape of your choice

1 1/4 cup sour cream

1 cup cottage cheese

1/3 cup onion, minced

Salt and pepper to taste

1/3 cup bread crumbs

Butter for the casserole dish

Method

Cook the noodles. Drain them and set them aside.

Cook the bacon until it is crisp. Drain it on paper towels. Crumble the bacon and set it aside.

Preheat the oven to 350°F.

Mix the cooked noodles, sour cream, cottage cheese, bacon pieces and onion. Season it all with salt and pepper and spoon it into a buttered casserole dish. Sprinkle the top of the casserole with the bread crumbs.

Bake for about 30 minutes.

Turkey Stuffing with Sausage and Apple

Ingredients

5 tablespoons butter

2 onions, medium, chopped

2 cups apple, chopped

1 cup celery, chopped

1 pound breakfast sausage, loose or removed from
their casings

3 cups corn bread, stale, crumbled

3 cups French bread, stale, crumbled

3 cups sandwich bread, stale, crumbled

1 1/2 teaspoons thyme, dried

1 cup parsley, fresh, chopped

2 eggs, lightly beaten

Salt & pepper to taste

2 cups turkey broth, or chicken broth

Method

In a large skillet melt 3 tablespoons of butter over
medium heat. Add the onion and celery and cook,
stirring, for 4 to 5 minutes or until the vegetables
are softened. Transfer to a large mixing bowl.

In the same skillet add 2 tablespoons of butter. When melted, add the apple and cook, stirring, for 5 to 6 minutes or until light golden. Transfer to the mixing bowl with the onion.

In same skillet, add the sausage. Cook, stirring to break up the sausage, for 7 to 8 minutes or until lightly brown. Transfer the meat to paper towels to drain. Then add it to the mixing bowl with the other ingredients. Stir to combine it all together. Preheat oven to 350ºF.

Add the corn bread pieces, French bread, sandwich bread, thyme, parsley and eggs to the bowl and stir just to combine it all. Season with salt and pepper. Pour in enough broth to moisten the dressing but not enough to make it runny. Spoon the dressing into a 13"x9" (33x23 cm) baking dish. Bake in preheated 350ºF (180ºC) oven for 45 minutes or until the stuffing is firm to the touch.

Turkey Stuffing with Apple Cranberry

Ingredients

1 cup raisins

7 cups bread crumbs, or soft cubed bread

3/4 cup butter, melted

1 cup onion, chopped

1 clove garlic, chopped

1 cup celery, chopped

3 cups apples, tart, diced into small pieces

1 cup dried cranberries

1/4 cup parsley, finely chopped

1 1/2 teaspoons salt

1 teaspoon sage

1 teaspoon savory

Method

Place the raisins in boiling water for 5 minutes, then drain well. Add the raisins to the bread crumbs.

Meanwhile, sauté the onion, garlic and celery in the butter. Add these vegetables, including all of the melted butter to the raisin mixture, then add the remaining ingredients. Mix it all together well.

Italian Tomato Bread Soup

Ingredients

5 slices Italian bread, ideally stale, crusts removed

3 tablespoons olive oil, extra virgin

6 cloves garlic, minced

2 pounds plum tomatoes, ripe, peeled, seeded and juice reserved or 1 - 35 ounce can Italian plum tomatoes, diced and seeded, juices reserved

4 cups chicken stock, or vegetable stock

Salt and black pepper

10 fresh basil leaves

Olive oil, extra virgin, for drizzling

Method

Preheat the oven to 375°F (only if you are using fresher bread).

If the bread is stale, just set it aside. If it is fresh, arrange the bread slices on a baking sheet and toast until they are light golden brown. Watch carefully so they don't burn. Remove and set aside.

Heat the olive oil in a large pot over medium heat. Add the garlic and cook until it is golden, about 6 minutes.

Add the tomatoes and their juices to the pot. Bring to a boil, stirring occasionally. Add the toasted bread and stock and return to a boil. Season lightly with salt and pepper and adjust the level of heat to a simmer.

Cook, uncovered for about 40 minutes. After 30 minutes add the basil leaves. Whisk occasionally to break up the pieces of bread. Adjust the seasoning if needed.

Serve with extra virgin olive oil drizzled over.

Lemon Cauliflower Rice

Ingredients

1 cauliflower, cut into florets

1 tablespoon oil

1 onion, small, diced

1 clove garlic, chopped

1/2 lemon, large, juice and zest

1/4 cup parsley, chopped

Salt & pepper to your taste

Method

Rice the cauliflower by grating it on the larger hole of a grater or putting the pieces through a food processor.

Heat the oil in a large pan to medium heat. Add the onion and garlic and sauté for a few minutes until the onion is just becoming translucent.

Add the cauliflower and salt and pepper it to your taste. Cook, stirring occasionally, until the cauliflower rice is tender and just slightly golden brown. This will take about 7 or 8 minutes.

Add the lemon juice, lemon zest and parsley into the cauliflower rice. Stir to mix everything together well and serve.

Tomatoes Florentine

Ingredients

6 tomatoes

2 teaspoons olive oil

1 onion, small, finely chopped

1 clove garlic, minced

12 ounces frozen spinach, chopped, thawed & drained

Pulp that you have removed from the tomatoes, chopped

Salt & pepper to taste

For the Topping:

2 tablespoons dry bread crumbs, plain or Italian style

2 tablespoons fresh parsley, chopped

2 teaspoons Parmesan cheese, grated

Method

Preheat the oven to 400ºF.

Cut a slice from the top of each tomato. Carefully scoop out the tomato pulp to about halfway down the tomato.

In a skillet, add the olive oil, then stir in the chopped onion, tomato pulp and garlic. Cook over medium heat until they are all tender, then stir in the spinach and the salt and pepper to taste. Heat the mixture together, then spoon it equally into the tomatoes.

Arrange the tomatoes in an oven proof baking dish.

For the Topping:

Combine the bread crumbs, chopped parsley and Parmesan cheese to make the topping. Sprinkle the mixture over top of the tomatoes as in the image. Bake the tomatoes in a preheated 400ºF oven for 20 minutes or until the topping is browned a bit and the tomatoes are heated through.

Pesto Parsley Recipe

Ingredients

2 cups parsley, firmly packed

1/2 cup fresh basil

1/2 cup olive oil

2 cloves garlic, peeled and chopped

Salt and pepper to taste

1/4 cup pine nuts, walnuts or almonds, chopped

1/2 cup Parmesan cheese, ideally freshly grated

Method

Place all the ingredients except the cheese in a blender or food processor. Blend everything together at high speed until the mixture is smooth, stopping occasionally to scrape the sides with a spatula.

Mix in the cheese and serve or store.

Pineapple Rice

Ingredients

1 cup basmati rice

1 onion, small, chopped

2 red chilies, large, optional

4 spring onions, chopped

4 ounces pineapple, chopped

1/2 cup vegetables, (a mixture of peas, carrots, corn
or green beans)

2 tablespoons oil

2 cloves garlic, crushed

1 tablespoon Thai fish sauce

1 tablespoon soy sauce

1 tablespoon sugar, optional

Salt and pepper to your taste

Method

Cook rice in boiling salted water for 10 minutes.
Rinse well and then drain it well. Set the rice aside
to cool.

While the rice is cooking, chop the onion, chilies (discarding seeds), spring onions, vegetables and pineapple. Set them aside.

Partially cook the vegetables if you are using fresh. Heat the oil in a large nonstick frying pan. Fry the garlic and onions for 2 to 3 minutes. Add the vegetables, chilies and spring onions, then add the cooked rice, fish, soy sauce and sugar.

Cook, stirring for about five minutes or until the mixture is piping hot. Stir in the pineapple. Cook for another minute.

Season with salt and pepper and serve.

Ginger Sauce with Steamed Asparagus

Ingredients

1 pound asparagus, cleaned

For the Ginger Sauce:

1 tablespoon soy sauce

1 teaspoon sugar, (optional)

1 teaspoon fresh ginger, grated

1 teaspoon dark sesame oil

1/4 teaspoon hot pepper sauce

1 tablespoon vegetable oil

1 teaspoon sesame seeds, toasted (optional)

Method

Prepare the asparagus spears by cutting or breaking off the tough ends.

Steam the asparagus spears until they are just tender and bright green, about 2 to 3 minutes. Drain them immediately and place them in a dish that will allow you to add in the dressing and mix it.

While the asparagus is steaming, mix together the soy sauce and sugar in a small bowl. Whisk it until the sugar dissolves, then stir in the grated ginger, sesame oil and hot sauce (if you are using it). Whisk in the vegetable oil until the vinaigrette thickens slightly. Pour the vinaigrette over the asparagus and toss it all gently to combine.

Toast the sesame seeds by placing them in a dry frying pan and heating them just until they begin to change color.

Transfer the dressed asparagus to a serving platter and sprinkle it with the toasted sesame seeds as a garnish and for fantastic taste.

Gingered Bok Choy

Ingredients

1 piece fresh ginger, (4 inches), peeled and julienned (or grated)

1 clove garlic

1 teaspoon salt

2 1/2 pounds baby bok choy, rinsed and trimmed

2 tablespoons tamari sauce, or soy sauce

Sesame seeds, for garnish (optional)

Method

Place the ginger, salt, garlic and 1 cup of water in a large pot or place a bit of water in a steamer with the vegetables in it. Cover the pot and bring to a simmer over low heat. Add the bok choy and cook, covered, until it is tender, about 5 minutes.

Drain the bok choy, sprinkle with the tamari or soy sauce and mix it slightly to cover it all with the sauce. Transfer it to a warmed serving dish and serve sprinkled with the sesame seeds.

Sautéed Rapini Recipe

Ingredients

1 pound rapini

2 onions

3 cloves garlic

1 tablespoon red pepper flakes, or more if you want it spicier

2 tablespoons olive oil

2 tablespoons lemon juice

5 tablespoons Italian parsley, finely chopped

Salt and pepper to taste

3 tablespoons pine nuts

Method

Cut off and discard the tough bottom of the rapini stems (probably about 2 inches). Coarsely chop the rest or leave the stems long. Wash the rapini and dry it a bit.

Peel and slice the onions. Peel and dice the garlic.

Heat the oil in a large, heavy bottomed frying pan on medium low heat and add the rapini, onions, red pepper flakes and garlic. Cover the pan and cook for 25 minutes, stirring occasionally.

Add the lemon juice, parsley, salt and pepper. Place the mixture in a serving bowl or plate.

Toast the pine nuts in the hot pan until they are golden brown. Watch them carefully as they toast so the nuts don't burn.

Add the pine nuts to the rapini, reserving a few toasted pine nuts to add to the top to serve.

Roasted Vegetable Medley

Ingredients

1 cup carrots, thinly sliced

1 cup green beans, sliced

1 cup potatoes, diced

2 tomatoes, medium, quartered

1 yellow squash, small, sliced

1 zucchini, small, sliced

1 onion, medium, sliced

1 cup eggplant, sliced and unpeeled

1/2 cup red pepper, chopped

3 cloves garlic, crushed

1/4 cup parsley, chopped

Freshly ground black pepper to your taste

1 cup beef bouillon

1/4 cup vegetable oil

2 teaspoons salt, or to your taste

1/4 teaspoon tarragon

Sprigs of fresh thyme

1/2 bay leaf

Method

Mix the cleaned and cut vegetables and garlic together and place into a shallow baking dish, 13" x 9" x 2". Sprinkle parsley over the top and grind black pepper over all. At this point you can refrigerate the casserole until ready to bake it.

Preheat the oven to 350°F.

Pour bouillon into a small saucepan, then add oil, salt, tarragon, and bay leaf. Heat to boiling and correct seasoning if necessary. Pour over vegetables. Sprinkle the fresh thyme over the vegetables.

Cover the baking dish with aluminum foil or parchment paper and bake at for 1 to 1 1/2 hours or until the vegetables are just tender and are still colorful. Carefully stir the vegetables occasionally while cooking, but, to preserve their color, don't lift the cover off for long.

Leave the cover off for the last few minutes of cooking time if you want the juices to cook into the vegetables more.

Recommended Dukan Diet Soup Recipes

Orzo with Lemon Chicken Soup

Ingredients

1 tablespoon olive oil

 3 carrots, peeled and diced

Half of an onion, diced

3 cloves garlic, minced

8–10 cups chicken broth

1 cup whole wheat orzo

3-ish cups cooked chicken (I use shredded rotisserie chicken)

3 eggs

Juice of 3–4 lemons (about 1/2 cup)

A handful of fresh spinach

1 1/2 teaspoons salt

Lots of freshly ground pepper

As much fresh dill as you can handle

Method

Heat large soup pot over medium heat. Add the olive oil. Add the carrots, onion, and garlic. Sauté until fragrant and tender, about 10 minutes. (Be careful not to burn the garlic.)

Add the broth and bring to a simmer. Add the orzo and cook for a few minutes until softened. Stir in the chicken and remove from heat.

Whisk the eggs and lemon juice together in a small bowl. The idea here is to warm up the egg mixture slowly (without scrambling the eggs). Slowly add a scoop of the soup into the egg mixture. Then add your warmed egg mixture back to the soup pot – slowly, slowly, slowly, stirring constantly, until smooth and creamy.

Finish by stirring in your spinach, salt, pepper, and dill and adjust seasonings to taste!

Vegetable & Barley Bean Soup

Ingredients

2 cups onions, chopped

1 cup carrots, chopped

1 cup celery, chopped

6 cups water

3 bouillon cubes, vegetable

28 ounces canned diced tomatoes, undrained

14 ounces canned kidney beans, rinsed and drained

1 cup quick cooking barley

1 teaspoon garlic powder

3/4 teaspoon pepper

1 package spinach, 10 ounces, fresh

Method

In a large saucepan with a 1/2 teaspoon of oil (or a non-stick frypan) sauté the onions, carrots and celery over medium heat for about 8 minutes or until the onions are soft.

Add in the water, bouillon, tomatoes, beans, barley, garlic powder and pepper. Bring the mixture to boil. Reduce heat, cover and simmer for 20 to 25 minutes.

Add spinach, cover and simmer for 1 or 2 minutes more or until the vegetables are tender.

South-western Black Bean Soup

Ingredients

2 teaspoons olive oil

1 onion, small, chopped

3 garlic clove, chopped

2 teaspoons ground cumin

3 carrots, sliced

3 parsnips, sliced

6 cups boiling chicken broth, water or vegetable broth

1 can black beans, drained

Method

Heat oil in a non-stick skillet. Add onions and sauté until they are translucent. Add garlic and cumin and cook 3 minutes longer. Add carrots and parsnips and cook 3 minutes longer. Add boiling broth or water. Deglaze the pot by stirring up the small bits from the bottom of the pot.

Add black beans. Simmer for 1 hour.

Bouillabaisse Recipe

Ingredients

1/4 cup onions, finely chopped

4 leeks, white portions only, finely cut into julienned strips

4 tomatoes, medium size, skinned and diced

5 cloves garlic, minced

1 tablespoon fresh fennel, finely chopped

1/2 - 3/4 teaspoon saffron

2 bay leaves, pulverized

1 teaspoon orange rind, grated

2 tablespoons tomato paste

1/8 teaspoon celery seed

3 tablespoons parsley, chopped

1 teaspoon pepper, freshly ground

2 tablespoons salt

1/4 - 1/2 cup olive oil

4 pounds in total of very fresh fish and seafood, diced in 1 inch pieces, in combination: red snapper, halibut, pompano, sea perch, scallops; also 1 inch pieces of well-scrubbed lobster, whole shrimp, clams and mussels - all in the shell

2 1/2 cups fish stock, or water

8 - 3/4 inch thick slices of French bread

Garlic butter

Method

Heat the oil in a large casserole. Combine onions, leeks, tomatoes, garlic, fennel, saffron, bay leaves, orange rind, celery seed, parsley and pepper and cook in the heated oil until the vegetables are transparent.

Add the fish and cover with the stock or water.

Keep the heat high and boil for 15 to 20 minutes.

Adjust the seasoning to your taste.

Dry the bread in the oven and brush it with garlic

butter.

Carrot Moroccan Soup Recipe

Ingredients

2 tablespoons butter

1 cup onions, chopped

1 pound carrots, peeled and chopped

2 1/2 cups chicken, or vegetable broth

1 1/2 teaspoons cumin

1 tablespoon honey

1 teaspoon lemon juice

1/2 cup yogurt

Method

Cook the butter, onions, carrots and chicken broth together. When the vegetables are cooked, puree the soup, then whisk in the cumin, honey and lemon juice.

Cioppino Recipe

Ingredients

2 tablespoons olive oil

1 1/2 cups scallions, sliced, white portion only

2 cups green peppers, diced

1 1/2 cups onion, diced

1 1/4 cups fennel, diced

1 tablespoon garlic, minced

1 cup dry white wine

1 quart fish broth

8 cups plum tomatoes, chopped, peeled and seeded

1/2 cup tomato puree

2 bay leaves

1/2 teaspoon salt, or as needed

1/2 teaspoon black pepper, freshly ground

20 littleneck clams, scrubbed well

3 hard-shell crabs, steamed

20 shrimp, medium, peeled and deveined

1 1/4 pounds swordfish steaks, or halibut, diced

3 tablespoons basil, shredded

Method

Heat the oil in a soup pot over medium heat. Add the scallions, peppers, onion, and fennel. Cook, stirring occasionally, until the onion is translucent, 6 to 8 minutes.

Add the garlic and cook for another minute.

Add the white wine, bring to a boil, and cook until the volume of wine is reduced by about half, 4 to 6 minutes.

Add the fish broth, tomatoes, tomato puree, and bay leaves. Cover the pot and simmer the mixture slowly for about 45 minutes. Add a small amount of water, if necessary. Cioppino should be more of a broth than a stew.

Season to taste with the salt and pepper. Remove and discard the bay leaves. Add the clams and simmer for about 10 minutes. Discard any clams that do not open.

Separate the claws from the crabs and cut the bodies in half. Add the crab pieces, shrimp, and swordfish to the soup. Simmer until the fish is just cooked through, about 5 minutes.

Add the basil and adjust the seasoning to taste, if necessary. Serve in heated bowls or soup plates.

Cream of Corn Soup

Ingredients

2 1/2 cups corn, cut from the ear, simmered until tender in 1 cup milk (or 2 1/2 cups creamed style canned corn)

3 tablespoons butter

1/2 onion, medium, sliced

3 tablespoons flour

1 1/2 teaspoons salt

Pinch black pepper, freshly ground

Nutmeg, grated, optional

3 cups milk, or 2 1/2 cups milk and 1/2 cup cream

3 tablespoons parsley, or chives, chopped, optional

Method

If you are using fresh corn, simmer it in 1 cup of milk until it is tender.

Put the cooked or canned corn through a food mill, food processor or coarse sieve. Melt the butter. Simmer the onion in the butter, until soft. Stir in the flour, salt and pepper, a touch of nutmeg, the corn and the milk. Heat through.

Serve the soup sprinkled with chives or parsley.

Parmentier Potage

Ingredients

6-7 russet potatoes

2 turnips

1 - 2 carrots, shredded

8 cups water, or chicken or vegetable broth

Salt and pepper to taste

Method

Peel the potatoes and chop them into large chunks.

Do the same with the turnips, cutting them into large chunks.

Take russet potatoes, skinned and large chopped, put in 2 turnips, skinned and large chopped. Boil in the water or chicken broth until the vegetables are soft and then process with a hand mixer in the pot to soup consistency (or transfer in batches to a blender).

Add the shredded carrots and 1-1/2 sticks butter. Cook on low heat until the carrots are soft and all flavors are melded. Season to taste with salt and pepper.

Bisque Shrimp Recipe

Ingredients

1 1/2 pounds shrimp, cooked, deveined and with shells removed

6 tablespoons butter

2 tablespoons onion, grated

3 cups milk, warm

1 cup cream

Salt, if needed

1 pinch paprika, or freshly ground white pepper

1 pinch nutmeg

3 tablespoons sherry

2 tablespoons parsley, or chives

Extra fresh chives or chopped parsley for garnish

Method

Put the shrimp through a meat grinder or blender and grind.

Cook the butter and onion, covered, in the top of a double boiler over, not in, hot water, for 5 minutes. Add the ground shrimp and milk and cook for 2 minutes. Stir the cream in slowly. Heat, but do not boil. Add the remaining ingredients. Heat all for about 3-5 minutes without letting it come to a boil. Serve at once.

Garnish with chopped fresh chives or parsley.

Butternut Squash Spicy Soup

Ingredients

1 green chili, chopped

2 cloves garlic, chopped

1 butternut squash, peeled and cut into pieces

3 carrots, chopped

2 onions, chopped

3 1/4 cups chicken stock, or vegetable stock

Salt and pepper to taste

2 teaspoons coriander, ground

1 teaspoon nutmeg, ground

1/2 teaspoon turmeric, ground

2 1/2 teaspoons cinnamon, ground

1 teaspoon honey

1/2 cup cream, or Crème Fraishe

Fresh cilantro to garnish, optional

Method

Fry the chopped garlic and chili. Add the other chopped vegetables. Add ALL the seasonings except the fresh coriander. Cook for a few minutes for the vegetables to partly soften - keep stirring. Add the stock and leave to boil for approximately 20 - 30 minutes. Take the pot off the heat and blend the soup (using a hand blender or food processor) to create a creamy soup.

Add the cream and fresh coriander and serve.

Ginger Squash Creamy Soup Recipe

Ingredients

1 onion, small, chopped

1 tablespoon butter

1 pound butternut squash, cubed and seeded

2 to 3 cups chicken broth, or vegetable broth

1 tablespoon ginger, chopped fresh

Pinch salt to taste

1 cup milk, half and half cream, or milk substitute of your choice

Method

In a 3 quart saucepan, cook the onions in butter for 5 minutes or until they are tender. Add the squash, broth and ginger. Cook over medium heat for 12 to 15 minutes or until the squash is very tender.

Place the squash, broth, ginger and salt into a blender jar. Cover the jar with the lid and blend at medium high speed until the soup has reached perfect consistency. Add more broth if you want a thinner soup. Also, if you prefer, you can easily blend the soup using a hand blender.

Return the mixture to the saucepan. Stir in the cream and gently heat the soup. Do not let it boil once the cream has been added.

Strawberry Watermelon Soup

Ingredients

4 cups watermelon, chunks

1 pint strawberries

1/2 cup yogurt

1 lemon, or 2-3 tablespoons lemon juice

2 tablespoons sugar

Fresh mint, optional

Method

Hull the strawberries. Peel and seed watermelon, cut into thumb sized chunks.

Put watermelon and sugar into a blender and blend until smooth. Pour mixture into chilled bowl.

Juice the lemon. Blend strawberries in the blender and slowly add yogurt and lemon juice while blending. Pour into bowl with watermelon and stir well. Put into the fridge for at least 2 hours. Use the fresh mint to garnish.

Serve ice-cold.

Taco Soup Recipe

Ingredients

1 to 1 1/2 pounds ground beef

1/2 teaspoons garlic, chopped

1 onion, large, chopped

1 - 16 ounce can tomatoes

1 - 16 ounce can tomato sauce

1 - 4 ounce can green chiles, optional

2 cups salsa

1 can corn, kernels, with juices

1 - 16 ounce can pinto beans

1 - 16 ounce can kidney beans

1 package taco seasoning mix, or make your own.

3 cups water

Suggested garnishes:

1 tablespoon cheddar cheese, grated

1/4 cup taco chips

2 tablespoons sour cream

Method

Brown ground beef with onion and garlic. When well browned, add the remaining ingredients and simmer for 1 hour.

Serve topped with grated cheddar cheese, taco chips, and a dollop of sour cream.

Chilled Red Pepper Soup Recipe

Ingredients

2 tablespoons olive oil

1 red onion, small, chopped

3 cloves garlic, slivered

1 1/2 cups carrots, sliced

4 sweet red peppers, large, cut into chunks

1 red apple chopped, (either skin on or peeled is fine)

6 plum tomatoes, chopped

1 tablespoon paprika

1 tablespoon brown sugar, packed

1 teaspoon salt

1 teaspoon dried thyme

1 teaspoon marjoram

1/4 teaspoon ground allspice

1 pinch cayenne pepper

Black pepper to taste

2 tablespoons sherry wine vinegar, or cider vinegar

Method

In a large stockpot, heat the oil over medium high heat. Cook the onion, garlic and carrots, stirring for 3-4 minutes or until the onion is softened.

Add the red peppers and the apple. Cook, stirring often, for about 15 minutes or until softened. Add the tomatoes during the last 5 minutes and cook for 5-6 minutes or until the mixture is bubbling.

Add the seasonings - the paprika, sugar, thyme, marjoram, allspice, cayenne and black pepper. Cook for 3 minutes.

Add vinegar. Bring the soup back to a boil. Add 4 cups water and return to a boil, stirring. Reduce the heat to medium low, cover and cook for 30 to 40 minutes, or until the vegetables are very soft. Let the soup cool until it is not super-hot. Purée the mixture in a blender in batches or use a hand blender to purée the soup. Transfer the soup to a large bowl and refrigerate it until it is chilled.

Wonton Soup

Ingredients

For the Soup Broth:

2 pounds chicken bones

1 onion, small, quartered

1 carrot, medium, quartered

1 1/2 inches ginger, peeled and sliced

12 cups water

For the Wonton Wrappers:

2 cups flour

1 teaspoon salt

2 eggs

1/2 cup water, +1 tablespoon

For the Wonton Filling:

1/2 inch ginger, fresh, grated

2 Thai chilies, fresh small red, halved lengthwise

8 ounces ground pork

1 garlic clove, crushed

1 green onion, chopped finely

2 tablespoons water chestnuts, finely chopped

2 tablespoons coriander, fresh, finely chopped

1/2 teaspoon sesame oil

2 tablespoons Chinese cooking wine

1/4 cup soy sauce

2 teaspoons sugar

Method

For the Broth:

Combine the chicken bones, onion, carrot, water, the ginger and half of the chili in a large saucepan. Bring the mixture to a boil, reduce heat, and simmer, uncovered for about two hours or until the mixture is reduced by half. Strain the broth through a lined sieve or a colander into a large bowl and discard the solids.

(Note that the broth can be made ahead to this stage. Cover and refrigerate overnight or freeze it if you prefer.)

To Make the Wontons:

Mix the flour and salt in a medium bowl. Make a well in the center of the flour. Break the eggs into the well. With a fork, beat the eggs and water for about 10 times. Gently start to work the flour and salt from the side of the well into the egg mixture until a dough forms and becomes sticky and difficult to work with a fork. Once all of the flour is incorporated into the dough, let it rest for 10 about minutes.

Once it has rested, knead the dough until it is smooth and elastic. Cover and let rest for another 30 minutes.

Divide the dough into three equal portions. Place 2 portions in a plastic bag. On a floured surface, roll out the third portion almost paper thin to a diameter of 12" x 12". With a knife or pastry wheel, cut 16 3" squares for wontons skins or cut 6 inch squares for egg roll wrappers. Sprinkle a little cornstarch between the squares, stack and place in a plastic bag. Repeat with the remaining dough.

Makes 40 to 50 wonton skins or about 12 egg roll wrappers.

To Make the Wonton Filling:

Chop the remaining chili finely. Combine in a small bowl with the pork, garlic, onion, finely chopped water chestnuts, fresh coriander, sesame oil, 2 teaspoons of the wine, 1 teaspoon of the soy sauce, half of the sugar and the remaining ginger.

You can make the wontons in two ways:

Fill the center of the wrapper with 2 teaspoons to 1 tablespoon of the pork filling, fold it over and press down the edges to seal. Then take the folded edges by the corners and overlap them to form a little hat-like dumpling. Or;

Place 2 teaspoons to one level tablespoon of pork filling on the center of each wonton wrapper and brush around the edges with a little water, then gather the edges tightly around the filling and pinch them together firmly to seal the wonton. Repeat this process with the remaining pork filling and wonton wrappers.

Finishing the Soup:

Skim the fat from the surface of the broth and return the broth to a large saucepan if it has been stored. Add the remaining wine, remaining soy sauce and remaining sugar and bring to a boil. Add the wontons to the pot and cook, uncovered for about five minutes or until cooked through. Using a slotted spoon, transfer the wontons from the pan to bowls then ladle the broth into bowls.

Recommended Dukan Diet Dessert Recipes

Apricot Pie Recipe

Ingredients

1 homemade pie dough for a double crust pie

2 cups dried apricots

2 cups water

1/2 cup sugar

1 1/2 tablespoons cornstarch

1 Pinch salt

3 tablespoons butter, cut into pieces

Method

Preheat the oven to 425°F.

For the homemade pie dough crust: Roll both disks of pie dough out to a 1/8-inch thickness on a floured surface. Fit one of the dough disks into a 9-inch pie pan. Trim the overhang to be even with the top of the pie pan. Set the other rolled-out crust aside.

In a small saucepan, bring the apricots and the water to a boil. Cook for 10 minutes over low heat. Add the sugar and cook for another 5 minutes, stirring occasionally. Using a colander, drain the contents of the saucepan, reserving 1 cup of the juice. Set the apricots aside.

Pour the reserved apricot juice into a small saucepan and add the cornstarch. Add the salt and cook over medium heat until the mixture thickens, 2 to 3 minutes, and stirring frequently until the consistency is like gravy.

Arrange the drained apricots in the unbaked pie shell. Pour the thickened apricot juice over the apricots. Dot the top with the butter. Use some water to wet the rim of the bottom crust, which will help both crusts adhere together.

Cover with the top crust and crimp the top and the bottom together all the way around. Slit the top 3 times and flute the edges. Bake for 30 minutes. Cover the edges only with foil, if needed, after 20 minutes, to prevent browning.

Cool on a wire rack or windowsill until the pie is firm, about 45 minutes. Store any leftovers in a sealed cake safe.

Fudge Brownies Recipe

Ingredients

4 ounces unsweetened chocolate, baker's chocolate squares

1/2 pound butter, or margarine

2 1/2 cups sugar

1 cup flour

4 eggs

2 cups pecans, chopped, or walnuts

Method

Preheat the oven to 350ºF (325ºF if using a glass baking dish).

Melt the chocolate and butter or margarine in a heavy saucepan over low heat. Remove from the heat and stir in the remaining ingredients in order, one at a time (the eggs also go in one at a time). Pour the mixture into a 9"x13" pan that has been lined with foil and greased.

Bake for 20 to 25 minutes. Do not over bake - the center should still have slightly moist crumbs when tested with a toothpick inserted into the center of the brownies.

Cool thoroughly before cutting.

Butterscotch Brownies

Ingredients

2/3 cup butter, or margarine, softened

1 1/2 cups brown sugar, firmly packed

2 eggs

2 teaspoons vanilla

2 cups flour

1 teaspoon baking powder

1/4 teaspoon baking soda

1 teaspoon salt

6 ounces butterscotch chips

1/2 cup pecans, chopped

Method

Preheat oven to 350°F.

Cream the butter and add the brown sugar, beating well. Add the eggs and vanilla to the mixture, beating well. Combine the flour, baking powder, baking soda and salt. Add the dry ingredients to the creamed mixture, stirring well. Pour the batter into a greased 13x9x2 inch baking pan.

Sprinkle with the morsels and pecans. Bake for 30 minutes. Cool and cut into bars.

Cream Cheese Brownies

Ingredients

For the Brownies:

4 ounces unsweetened baking chocolate

1 cup butter, or margarine

2 cups sugar

2 teaspoons vanilla

4 eggs, large

1 1/2 cups all-purpose flour

1/2 teaspoon salt

1 cup nuts, coarsely chopped

For the Cream Cheese Filling:

16 ounces cream cheese, softened (2 - 8 ounce packages)

1/2 cup sugar

2 teaspoons vanilla

1 egg

Method

Heat the oven to 350°F. Grease the bottom and sides of a rectangular pan, 13x9x2 inches, with shortening or non-stick spray.

Melt the chocolate and butter in a 1-quart saucepan over low heat, stirring frequently. Let it cool.

Beat the cream cheese filling ingredients together until smooth and set aside.

Beat together the cooled chocolate mixture, sugar, vanilla and eggs in a large bowl with an electric mixer on medium speed for 1 minute, scraping the bowl occasionally.

Beat in the flour and salt on low speed for 30 seconds, scraping the bowl occasionally. Beat on medium speed for 1 minute. Stir in the nuts. Spread half of the batter (2 1/2 cups) in the pan. Spread the cheesecake filling over the batter. Carefully spread the remaining brownie batter over the cream cheese filling.

You can bake it as is or create the pretty design you see in the picture. To do that, take a butter knife and insert it into the layers of batter. Swirl the knife a bit so that the batters mix just a bit into a swirl pattern as in the image.

Bake in an oven preheated to 350°F for 45-50 minutes or until a toothpick inserted in the center comes out clean. Cool the cheesecake brownies in the pan on a wire rack.

Coconut Macaroon and Chocolate Brownie Recipe

Ingredients

4 ounces unsweetened chocolate

3/4 cup butter

2 3/4 cups sugar, divided

5 eggs, divided

1 cup flour, + 2 tablespoons, divided

2 cups almonds, toasted and chopped

8 ounces cream cheese, softened

2 cups sweetened coconut, flaked

Method

Preheat oven to 350ºF.

Melt unsweetened chocolate and butter over low heat until the butter is melted. (You can also do this in the microwave for 2 minutes on medium power). Stir until completely smooth.

Stir in 2 cups of the sugar and 3 eggs. Stir in 1 cup flour and half of the chopped almonds. Spread the mixture in a greased and foil lined 9"x13" baking pan.

Beat the cream cheese with the remaining sugar, eggs and flour until smooth. Stir in remaining almonds and the coconut. Spread over the brownie batter.

Bake 35 to 40 minutes or until a toothpick inserted into the center comes out almost clean.

Chocolate Brownies with Raspberry Filling

Ingredients

1 cup unsalted butter

5 ounces unsweetened chocolate, chopped

2 cups sugar

4 eggs

2 teaspoons vanilla extract

1 1/4 cups flour

1 teaspoon baking powder

1/2 teaspoon salt

1 cup walnuts, toasted and chopped

1/2 cup raspberry preserves

Method

Melt the butter and chocolate in a heavy saucepan over low heat, stirring constantly until smooth. Remove from the heat. Whisk in the sugar, eggs and vanilla. Mix the flour, baking powder and salt in a small bowl. Add to the chocolate mixture and whisk to blend. Stir in the nuts.

Pour 2 cups of batter into a buttered 13x9 inch pan (or use the specialty brownie pan shown below for lots of edges). Freeze until firm, about 10 minutes. Spread the preserves over the frozen batter. Spoon the remaining batter over the preserves. Let stand for 20 minutes at room temperature to thaw.

Bake at 350°F for 35 minutes or until tester comes out clean. Transfer to a rack to cool.

Banana Cream Pie Recipe

Ingredients

3/4 cup sugar

1/3 cup all-purpose flour, or 3 tablespoons cornstarch

1/4 teaspoon salt

2 cups milk

3 egg yolks, slightly beaten

2 tablespoons butter

1 teaspoon vanilla

3 to 4 bananas, sliced

1 pastry crust, 9", baked

Meringue, made from the leftover egg whites, optional

Method

Combine sugar, cornstarch, and salt in a saucepan. Add milk gradually. Cook, stirring constantly, over medium heat till bubbly. Cook and stir an additional 2 minutes and remove from burner.

Stir small amount of hot mixture into egg yolks, immediately add egg yolk mixture to hot mixture and cook for 2 minutes, stirring constantly. Remove from heat.

Add butter and vanilla and stir till smooth.

Slice 3-4 bananas into the cooled baked pastry shell. Top with pudding mixture and spread meringue or fresh whipped cream (if desired) on top of the pie. Cool.

Blueberry Pie Recipe

Ingredients

4 cups blueberries, fresh, or frozen if that is all you have

1 tablespoon lemon juice

1 Pastry for double-crust 9 inch pie

1 cup sugar

1/3 cup flour

1/4 teaspoon ground cinnamon

1/8 teaspoon ground nutmeg

1 dash ground cloves

2 tablespoons butter, or margarine

1 egg yolk

1 tablespoon water

Method

Preheat the oven to 400°F.

Place the blueberries in a bowl and sprinkle them with lemon juice.

Roll half of the crust to about 1/8" in thickness and fit it into a 9" pie plate.

Combine the sugar, flour and spices and stir well. Add the flour mixture to the berries, stirring well to mix it all in. Pour the berry mixture into the pastry lined pie plate. Dot the filling with butter.

Roll out the remaining crust to 1/8" thickness. Cover the pie with the crust. Trim the pastry around the edge of the pie pan. Seal and flute the edges. Cut slits in the crust top for steam to escape.

Combine the egg yolk and water. Lightly brush the pastry top with the egg mixture.

Bake at 400°F for 40-45 minutes or until golden brown. Cool before serving.

Buttermilk Pie Recipe

Ingredients

Cowboy Piecrust:

1 1/3 cups all-purpose flour, plus 1-2 tablespoons

1/2 teaspoon salt

1/2 teaspoon ground cinnamon

1/2 teaspoon sugar

1/2 cup vegetable shortening, chilled

3 tablespoons cold water

Buttermilk Pie Filling:

2 cups sugar

2 tablespoons cornmeal

5 eggs, beaten

2/3 cup buttermilk

2 tablespoons butter, melted, room temperature

1 teaspoon vanilla extract

2 teaspoons lemon rind, minced

3 teaspoons lemon juice

Method

For the crust, mix the flour, salt, cinnamon and sugar in a medium size bowl. Cut in the shortening using a pastry blender or 2 knives, until all the flour is blended in and the mixture consists of pea-size bits. Sprinkle the mixture with water, 1 tablespoon at a time. Toss lightly with a fork until the dough forms a ball.

Work the dough, pressing between your hands to form a 5-6 inch pancake. If the dough seems too sticky, wrap in plastic and refrigerate for 20-30 minutes. Dust the dough lightly with 1-2 extra tablespoons of flour.

Roll the dough in a circle between 2 sheets of waxed paper on a slightly dampened countertop.

Peel off the top sheet of waxed paper, then trim the dough so that it has 1 inch lapping over the edges of a 9 inch pie plate. Turn the dough over onto the pie plate, pull the waxed paper away. And press the pastry to fit the pan. Fold the edge of the pastry under and flute the edges or press with fork tines. For the pie, preheat the oven to 350°F.

In a bowl, combine the sugar and cornmeal. Add the eggs and buttermilk, mixing well. Add the butter, vanilla, lemon rind and lemon juice. Mix until blended. Pour into the pie shell and bake for 45 minutes. Or just until beginning to brown on top.

Moist Carrot Cake Recipe

Ingredients

3/4 cup sugar

1 cup vegetable oil

4 eggs

1 cup white flour

1 cup whole wheat flour

1 1/2 teaspoons baking soda

1 teaspoon salt

2 teaspoons cinnamon

2 cups carrots, grated

1 1/2 cups apples, peeled and grated

1 cup raisins

1/2 cup walnuts

Cream Cheese Icing:

4 ounces cream cheese

1/4 cup butter, softened

1 cup icing sugar

Method

Mix together the sugar, oil and eggs until the mixture is slightly thickened. Sift the flours together with the soda, salt and cinnamon.

Add the flour mixture to the egg mixture. Add the carrots, apples, raisins and walnuts. Stir until evenly mixed.

Bake in a greased and floured pan, 9"x13"x2" or a Bundt type pan or two round cake pans. Bake at 350ºF for about 35 minutes if using the 13" long pan.

Always check for doneness by piercing the center of the cake with a toothpick. If it comes out clean, it's done.

If you use the round cake pans, check for doneness about 5 to 10 minutes earlier as they are smaller and you don't want to over bake the cake. On the other hand, if you are baking the cake in a Bundt style cake pan check your cake carefully for doneness after 40 minutes and leave it in 5 minutes longer if you need to.

Let the cake cool and ice with the cream cheese icing below. Blend all of the icing ingredients together and spread over the cooled cake.

Almond and Coconut Balls

Ingredients

1/2 cup almond meal

1/2 cup coconut flakes

1/4 cup sesame seeds

1 cup walnuts, chopped, cashews or pistachios

16 ounces almond butter, or cashew butter, softened

3 tablespoons tahini

1/2 teaspoon vanilla extract

8 drops Stevia, liquid or equivalent in dry Stevia.

4 tablespoons walnuts, seeds or cocoa powder for coating.

Method

Put the almond meal, coconut flakes, sesame seeds, nuts, nut butter, tahini, vanilla and Stevia in a bowl. Mix it all together with a wooden spoon until well combined.

Using your hands, take about a tablespoonful (not more or the balls will be too large) of the mixture and roll it into a ball. Roll the ball in the coating of your choice, coating the balls well all over. You may need to press the balls into the seeds or nuts well to make sure they stick. Repeat until you have used all of the almond mixture. You should end up with 14 to 16 medium size balls.

Place the balls on a flat tray in the refrigerator to firm up. Store the coconut balls in the refrigerator, well wrapped, until you are ready to serve them. Take them out to soften about 30 minutes before you want to eat them.

Almond Cookie Recipe

Ingredients

2 cups ground almonds

3/4 cup sugar

1 egg white

1/4 teaspoon almond extract

18 pecan halves, optional

Method

Preheat the oven to 350°F.

Place the ground almonds and sugar in a medium bowl. Using a whisk, beat the egg white and almond extract in a small bowl until frothy and beginning to hold its shape. Do not beat it into a hard meringue, but until just about the time you begin to get soft peaks.

Gradually beat the egg mixture into the ground almonds and sugar until the mixture becomes a fairly stiff paste. You may not need all the egg white. Make sure that you do not make the mixture too soft.

Drop the cookie mixture by the tablespoonful, 1 inch apart on a baking sheet that is lined with a non-stick liner or baking parchment. Flatten the mixture slightly with a fork dipped in water or to keep a smoother surface, use your fingers dipped in a bit of water. If you wish, gently press a pecan half into the center of the cookie.

Bake for 10-12 minutes at 350°F, or until just set, but still soft inside. Do not allow the macaroons to go brown, as they should be fairly pale. Transfer the cookies to a wire rack and leave them to cool until they are firm before removing them from the baking sheet. Place them on a rack to let them cool completely. Store in an airtight container.

Makes 16-18 cookies, but the recipe can easily be doubled.

Eggplant Dip Recipe

Ingredients

1 eggplant, large

1 clove garlic, large, minced

1 tomato, large, peeled & chopped

1 stalk celery, finely chopped

1/4 cup green pepper, or red, finely chopped

3 green onions, finely chopped

1 tablespoon lemon juice

2 teaspoons vegetable oil, or olive oil

1/2 teaspoon salt

1/4 teaspoon freshly ground pepper

Method

Preheat the oven to 400ºF (200ºC).

Poke the eggplant in several places with fork. Place it on a baking sheet and bake in the preheated oven for 45 minutes or until soft, turning once or twice during baking. Let the eggplant cool, then peel it and chop finely.

Meanwhile, sauté the garlic, celery, green pepper and tomatoes in a bit of oil for 4 or 5 minutes or until they soften. Add the chopped green onions in the last minute of cooking.

In a mixing bowl, combine the eggplant, onions, garlic, tomato, celery and green pepper and toss to mix them all together. Add the lemon juice, oil, salt and pepper. Stir to mix well. Cover and refrigerate the dip for at least 1 hour before serving for the flavors to meld.

Tomato Salsa

Ingredients

10 cups tomatoes, chopped, I use canned diced

5 cups green peppers, yellow, red or orange, chopped

2 1/2 cups jalapeno, chopped, or any hot pepper of your choice

5 cups onion, diced

1 tablespoon pickling salt

1/2 cup garlic, minced

1 1/4 cup pure apple cider vinegar

Method

Put all in a heavy bottom Dutch oven and heat until simmering, let simmer for about one hour. Pour hot into sterilized jars and seal.

Vietnamese Spring Rolls

Ingredients

2 tablespoons soy sauce

2 tablespoons Asian chili sauce, sweet

1/2 teaspoon sesame oil, toasted

1/2 teaspoon rice vinegar

1/2 teaspoon garlic, minced

1/2 teaspoon pickled ginger, finely chopped

1/4 teaspoon ginger root, minced

2 cups baby bok choy, shredded

3/4 cup asparagus, julienned blanched, (see Tips, below)

3/4 cup carrots, julienned, peeled

1/2 cup English cucumber, julienned

1/4 cup mango, julienned

1/4 cup peanuts, finely chopped, toasted

8 - 10- inch rice paper, egg roll wrappers

3 cups hot water

Method

In a bowl, combine soy sauce, chili sauce, oil, vinegar, garlic, pickled ginger and minced ginger.

For the rolls: In another bowl, combine bok choy, asparagus, carrots, cucumber, mango and peanuts.

Add 2 tablespoons of the dressing and toss well.

Divide the vegetables into 8 equal portions.

Working with only one rice paper at a time, submerse the sheet in hot water until pliable, which will take about 30 seconds. Place it on a work surface.

Spread one-portion of the vegetable mixture in a strip across the rice paper wrapper about one-third away from the edge closest to you, leaving about 1 inch (2.5 cm) on either side. Fold the edge closest to you over the filling and pull gently toward you to encase the filling. Fold the sides toward the middle, then continue to roll up tightly.

Place the rolls under a damp cloth to stay moist because the wrappers tend to dry out quickly. Serve the rolls immediately with the dipping sauce below, if using, or refrigerate for up to 1 hour.

To make a wonderful dipping sauce:

In a small ramekin, combine the remaining dressing with 1/4 cup soy sauce and 1 tablespoon coarsely chopped peanuts.

Chapter 4:   Adjusting Your Lifestyle to Better Results

aking changes to one's way of life is crucial if one wants to keep the weight off and improve their health and wellness in general. By making these adjustments, you may establish and maintain healthy routines that help you maintain a healthy weight and lead a more satisfying and well-rounded life.

Making healthy eating a top priority is one of the most important changes you can make to your lifestyle if you want to keep the weight off. Eating a diet rich in plant-based foods, lean proteins, whole grains, and healthy fats while cutting less on sugar, processed foods, and bad fats is part of this. One way people may make sure they're getting all the nutrients they need without going overboard on calories is by eating whole meals and controlling their portions.

One of the most important things you can do for your health is to exercise regularly. Regular exercise, whether it's brisk walking, running, cycling, swimming, or strength training, boosts metabolism, burns calories, and improves health and fitness. The key to long-term motivation and physical activity is finding things that you like and can keep up with.

Lifestyle changes include eating better, exercising more, and controlling your emotions, stress, and sleep habits. Gaining weight and other health problems can be caused by hormones that regulate hunger and metabolism being disrupted by chronic stress and inadequate sleep. Incorporating stress-reduction practices like yoga, deep breathing, meditation, or mindfulness into your routine and sticking to a regular sleep pattern will greatly benefit your health and weight maintenance efforts.

One of the most significant lifestyle changes you can make to keep the weight off is to surround yourself with encouraging people. A great way to stay motivated, accountable, and encouraged is to surround yourself with others who share your health objectives, whether that's family, friends, or support groups. A more pleasant and encouraging environment at home and in the workplace can help people maintain their healthy habits and triumph over obstacles.

In the grand scheme of things, making changes to one's way of life is essential for sustaining weight reduction and improving one's health in general. Managing one's weight and achieving a balanced lifestyle may be accomplished by the adoption of good eating habits, frequent physical activity, stress management skills, and supportive situations.

What Kind of Exercise Should I Do?

To maximize weight reduction and general health and fitness, it is recommended to incorporate appropriate workouts into each phase of the

Dukan Diet. Participants may find it helpful to concentrate on low-impact activities like walking, swimming, or cycling during the Attack Phase, the initial stage of the program. You may burn calories and aid weight reduction with these exercises without overstressing your body, which may be adapting to a new diet.

In the Cruise Phase, when participants are able to eat a wider variety of foods and avoid starchy vegetables, they may find that they have greater stamina to exercise at a moderate intensity. To enhance cardiovascular fitness, calorie expenditure, and assist ongoing weight reduction, try jogging, aerobics courses, or the gym's cardio equipment.

Participants can keep up with a variety of workouts to help them maintain their weight and general health throughout the Consolidation Phase, which entails eating carbs and fats again while still focusing on lean protein and veggies. Weightlifting and other forms of strength training can aid in the development of lean muscle mass, which in turn increases metabolic rate and facilitates the maintenance of a healthy weight over the long run.

During the Stabilization Phase, which marks the beginning of a healthy lifestyle habits that will last a lifetime, participants can keep doing a variety of activities to maintain their weight, including cardio, strength training, flexibility, and balance. Supporting general health, increasing fitness levels, and preventing long-term weight regain are all goals of this holistic approach to fitness.

When it comes down to it, everyone's fitness level, taste, and objectives determine which workouts are best for each stage of the Dukan Diet. To support weight loss or maintenance efforts and promote general health and well-being, it is important to pick activities that are pleasant, sustainable, and suitable for one's current fitness level.

Common Challenges Peculiar to the Dukan Diet

Although many have found success on the Dukan Diet, which provides a systematic method to losing weight, there are a few distinct obstacles that dieters may face.

The Attack Phase, in particular, requires the consumption of only meals high in pure protein, which might be a struggle. The other stages are just as rigorous. Diet long-term adherence may be challenging for certain people because to feelings of deprivation and boredom brought on by this limitation. Furthermore, not everyone can maintain the fast weight reduction that occurs during the Attack Phase, which can result in rebound weight gain when regular eating habits are restored.

Planning and preparing meals, particularly for those with dietary limitations or preferences, can be a struggle during the beginning phases of the

Dukan Diet due to the restricted selection of foods that are allowed. Although there is considerable leeway in the plan's food selections, some people may find the emphasis on lean protein and non-starchy veggies to be too much, and end up bored or unhappy with the diet.

When you're out to eat with friends or at a gathering where food options are restricted, the Dukan Diet's stringent rules and regulations could be a problem. People on the diet may experience feelings of loneliness or exclusion due to the pressure to follow the rules to the letter, even when doing so would be difficult or impossible.

Some people also worry about the long-term implications of the Dukan Diet, especially because of how much animal protein it requires and since it cuts out whole food categories like carbs and fats. The diet's effects on long-term health and durability are still up for question, however it may cause quick weight loss in the short-term.

While many have found success on the Dukan Diet, which provides an organized approach to weight management, some may find it difficult to stick to the program over the long term due to the difficulties it brings. Before starting the Dukan Diet or any other weight reduction program, it's wise to evaluate one's own preferences, lifestyle variables, and possible health consequences.

What You Can do to Achieve Your Goals

A mix of tactics and mental adjustments is needed to overcome the obstacles of the Dukan Diet and make it more sustainable and pleasurable in the long run.

One option is to become inventive with meal planning so that you may still adhere to the diet's rules while still enjoying a range of foods. To make protein-rich dishes more appetizing and pleasurable to consume, try experimenting with various seasonings, herbs, and spices. Meals may be made more visually appealing and nutritionally gratifying by adding a range of non-starchy veggies.

Making meals in advance is another way to make sure you stick to the diet plan even when you have a lot on your plate with social commitments and work. You may save time and make it simpler to keep to your diet, even on busy days, by batch cooking protein-rich dishes and veggies. One further thing that can help people remain on track when they go out to restaurants or social gatherings is to bring snacks or portable protein sources.

To get through the tough times on the Dukan Diet, it might help to surround yourself with supportive people, whether that's in real life or online. Staying on track and overcoming challenges might be simpler when you connect with people who are also following the diet or have similar health objectives. They can offer support, hold you accountable, and motivate you.

Another way to keep yourself motivated and devoted to your weight reduction objectives is to think about the long-term benefits of the Dukan Diet. These include better health, more energy, and higher self-confidence. Diet success is more likely to last when people stop thinking of it as a quick cure and start seeing it as a way of life change.

Maintaining success on the Dukan Diet calls for an optimistic outlook, some pliability, and the ability to roll with the punches. Individuals may accomplish their weight reduction objectives on the Dukan Diet in a sustainable and pleasurable manner by being innovative, planning ahead, seeking help, and concentrating on the long-term advantages.

Chapter 5:   Conclusion

The Dukan Diet provides a systematic way to lose weight, and it works for a lot of people. The goal of the program is to encourage fast weight reduction with no negative effects on muscle mass or general health by focusing on low-carb, high-protein meals and by implementing distinct phases with clear instructions. The Dukan Diet is successful, but it comes with its own share of problems, including a lack of variety in the food you may eat, restrictions on how you can interact socially, and worries about the diet's impact on your health in the long run.

Finding new methods to spice up meals, making a game plan, reaching out to friends and family for support, and keeping an eye on the big picture of the diet's advantages are all ways that people may overcome these obstacles. People may successfully lose weight on the Dukan Diet and keep it off for good if they go into it with an optimistic outlook, a little bit of flexibility, and a readiness to adjust.

Maintaining a healthy weight requires a commitment to a balanced diet, frequent exercise, stress management, and surrounding yourself with positive people. Individuals may lose weight, keep it off, and enhance their health and wellness for good by making simple changes to their everyday routine.

Though not everyone will find success on the Dukan Diet, everyone can learn a lot about healthy eating and portion control from the program's systematic approach. Individuals may accomplish long-term success and live a balanced, satisfying life by adopting a holistic perspective on health and wellbeing.